D1112543

The Briles Report
on Women in
Healthcare

The Briles Report On Women in Healthcare

Changing Conflict to Collaboration in a Toxic Workplace

Judith Briles

Jossey-Bass Publishers • San Francisco

Substantial discounts on bulk quantities of Jossey-Bass books are available to corporations, professional associations, and other organizations. For details and discount information, contact the special sales department at Jossey-Bass Inc., Publishers. (415) 433-1740; Fax (415) 433-0499.

For international orders, please contact your local Paramount Publishing International office.

Manufactured in the United States of America. Nearly all Jossey-Bass books, jackets, and periodicals are printed on recycled paper that contains at least 50 percent recycled waste, including 10 percent postconsumer waste. Many of our materials are also printed with vegetable-based ink; during the printing process these inks emit fewer volatile organic compounds (VOCs) than petroleum-based inks. VOCs contribute to the formation of smog.

Library of Congress Cataloging-in-Publication Data

Briles, Judith.
   The Briles report on women in healthcare : changing conflict to collaboration in a toxic workplace / Judith Briles, — 1st ed.
     p.   cm. — (The Jossey-Bass social and behavioral science series)
   Includes bibliographical references and index.
   ISBN 1-55542-671-9
   1. Women in medicine. 2. Work environment. 3. Work—
—Psychological aspects. I. Title. II. Series.
R692.B66 1994
158'.26'082—dc20   94-12540
                                                               CIP

FIRST EDITION
HB Printing 10 9 8 7 6 5 4 3 2 1   *Code 9472*

Contents

To Sylvia Eaton, RN,
whose tenacity saved my life

Preface

We all know it exists. Most of us have experienced it. At least some of us practice it. Sabotage, backstabbing, backbiting, vicious gossip, and other undermining behaviors are alive and well in the workplace. That is the problem. Exposing these toxic behaviors and outlining how we can stop them is the purpose of this book.

For many years, I have been asking women and men to tell me about their experiences with sabotage at work. My primary interests are in learning more about women's experiences and how women stop destructive patterns. What I have found as I criss-cross the country, speaking to approximately 40,000 women a year, is that women working in a variety of professions consistently report that they have been undermined more by other women than by men. They also report a substantial increase in the amount of sabotage.

Why might this be so? I believe that sabotaging is a learned behavior, in itself a misplaced attempt at workplace survival, not a genetic trick of nature. I also believe that with education, awareness, and commitment, sabotage can change. Once sabotage ends and real support systems begin, women and men benefit emotionally, physically, and financially. Their co-workers do likewise.

In this work, I turn specifically to women working in healthcare, one of the most female-dominated work settings in America. The healthcare industry will provide over 10 million jobs by the year 2000. Over 70 percent of those positions—7 million jobs—will be held by women. Over 2.5 million nursing positions will be available, with 93–95 percent filled by women. In dentistry, staff and hygienists will fill an estimated 900,000 jobs. What might a look inside the healthcare industry tell us about surviving and thriving in any work setting? Read on.

The Origins of This Work

In the winter of 1992, I had just completed the second presentation of a two-part program at the Glens Falls Hospital, in Glens Falls, New York. After the evening program, several organizers and participants and I met at a restaurant in neighboring Sarasota Springs. The house specialty was pizza. It was delicious, but the conversation that followed was even better.

My dinner companions held various positions within their hospital. They were clinical specialists, staff nurses, and nurse executives. While sharing food and stories that evening, Kathleen Kennedy, vice president for nursing care, encouraged me to undertake the study that is the basis for this report. The health field would provide quite a laboratory, we reasoned, when so many employees—especially those at the bottom rungs of the career ladders—are female. Here—inside our hospitals, clinics, doctors' and dentists' offices, and the like—how did women (and men) really work together? Would they support each other because they saw themselves as caretakers with a vital—indeed, a life-and-death—public trust? Would the service aspect of working in healthcare make a difference? Would levels of conflict that I had found in other work settings be repeated in healthcare?

Would women workers in healthcare undermine each other more than my earlier work in the generic workplace had found? Several of the women sitting around the table eating pizza and talking about their work experiences that night in 1992 said they thought that backstabbing and undermining behavior had increased over the past few years. Terms like *abuse* and *assault* were used openly and freely. Neither of those words had surfaced in my previous interviews or surveys. I made a note to ask other women about this, too.

That note was the seed for this report, and as I left my colleagues in New York that night, I was determined to begin a new nationwide study of working women, one focused on healthcare professionals and drawing from my earlier work. Over the next year, I continued to talk and listen to women in healthcare. I conducted interviews, a survey, and numerous workshops.

The results of my study are the subject of this work. To offer a quick overview, let me say that I found sabotage had increased, and that there were basically two reasons for it: first, women were more aware of what sabotaging and undermining behavior is and were willing to identify it; and, second, women are the least likely to have seniority or authority in their workplaces, and so any reorganizing or downsizing will be likely to affect them first. The second part of the book offers tools and strategies to help stop sabotage and enable women to work together in a healthy environment.

Audience

This book is written for several audiences, including men. Women workers in all fields will recognize themselves and their co-workers. Women who work in nursing, medicine, healthcare administration, medical insurance, health centers, hospitals, dentistry, and pharmaceuticals may laugh, cry, or get angry at the familiarity of the stories recorded in this work.

Women and men who read this work will want to change their workplaces—for themselves and for others. They will be able to recognize sabotaging and other unacceptable behaviors in others (and sometimes in themselves) and identify appropriate ways to change destructive interactions. It is my hope that the readers of this work will truly believe that their voices do count and that together they can transform their toxic workplaces into thriving communities.

Acknowledgments

While it is an author with a vision who conceives a book, that book cannot be delivered without the help of a birthing team. Begun in Glens Falls, New York, and developed in Denver, this book was born under the able care of the Jossey-Bass team in San Francisco. My editor, Rebecca McGovern, immediately saw the book's potential. She was a pleasure to work with. I thank her for her skills in maintaining my message as she helped trim and revise the original manuscript. Margaret Sebold brought her marketing savvy to the table and was always open to ideas. Xenia Lisanevich and Pamela Berkman did the final shaping, working closely with everyone on the team. I look forward to working with each again, and am grateful for their humor and dedication.

The hundreds of women who work in the healthcare field have been generous with their time and insights beyond anything I imagined. I thank the survey respondents and the more than 100 women who agreed to be interviewed. Their voices make this book. All names have been changed to respect these women's requests and the need for confidentiality. My cronies, Steve Achtenhagen, Stephanie West Allen, Pat Burns, Susan Dolkas, Denise Fonseca, Patricia Fripp, Ed Greif,

Jaclyn Kostner, Susan RoAne, Nicole Schapiro, and Carol Ann Wilson have been my cheerleaders for years. Edward De Croce, who took the jacket photo, has a terrific eye and brings out the best in any of his subjects. Thank you all for being there.

And of course, none of my books are created without the support of my staff. John Maling transferred data from the surveys to computer and tallied results; Becky Brandt transcribed hundreds of hours of interviews and my own tapes to deliver the working manuscript and its multiple revisions; Sheryl Briles read and reread each revision, never holding back her comments and recommendations. I thank them all.

Part One

The Survey Speaks

1

What Women Say
About Sabotage

I didn't want to believe it was happening. It was one of those times in my life that I didn't listen to myself. I kept pushing it down, saying, "This isn't true. It can't be happening. She's really not like this." When I finally opened my eyes and ears, I found that everything she did was for her own benefit. There really wasn't any effort to do anything as a team member or a partner.

Woman to Woman, a study I published in 1987, produced a major brouhaha in working women's circles. The results showed that when it comes to unethical, undermining, sabotaging behavior, men do not discriminate: they behave unethically toward both sexes, in equal measure. Their style of being unethical is also different from women's: men are more overt, and very direct; they let you know if they intend to undermine you.

But if a woman is going to be unethical and unsupportive, and if she displays other types of sabotaging behavior, her target is more likely to be another woman, and her style is likely to be covert. Sometimes her target doesn't even know where the sabotage has come from.

When these results were released to the media, such women's

magazines as *New Woman, Working Woman, McCall's, Redbook, Family Circle, Ladies' Home Journal,* and *Cosmopolitan* ignored these findings. *Glamour* was different. The editors of *Glamour* decided to query their readers in a survey of their own. I supplied my data, the results, and the questions asked. They asked similar questions of their readers. *Glamour's* findings were published in June 1988. The editors were surprised. I wasn't. *Glamour's* readers agreed with my study. With another source confirming my results, I felt that the problem of women's undermining other women would move from being a taboo topic to being one that could be addressed, discussed, and resolved.

Survey Respondents

My 1987 survey respondents had come from the general workplace—corporations, associations, institutions, academia. Some of them (nurses and doctors) had come from healthcare. Others worked for companies that manufactured products used in healthcare. But in the 1993 survey, conducted for this book, the respondents came solely from the healthcare field.

Questionnaires were sent to directors of women's centers, vice presidents for nursing, and educational departments at randomly selected hospitals. Each questionnaire was accompanied by a cover letter. Survey recipients were provided with Webster's definition of the term *unethical behavior,* which they were free to interpret however they saw fit. Surveys were also distributed at the annual meeting of the National Association of Women Health Professionals (NAWHP), a not-for-profit organization formed in 1987 and representing seven hundred members in the United States and Canada. In fact, NAWHP was selected as the primary locus of survey distribution, since its membership is diverse and consists of program directors, hospital administrators, nurses, physicians, marketing and planning directors, policy analysts, and educational professionals. The common link is the fact that all members work in the field of women's healthcare. NAWHP's members and the exhibitors at its annual meeting represent a cross-section of predominantly women in the healthcare industry.

Of the 1,000 surveys sent out, 229 were returned by the cutoff date. An additional 5 percent were received after the cutoff date but were not included statistically; in a postevaluation, they revealed the same types of responses as in the surveys received before the cutoff date. Of the 229 surveys, 5 were returned by men. The largest number of responses from individual states came from Colorado, Iowa, Florida, Louisiana, Michigan, New Hampshire, and Ohio.

The participants consisted of 98 percent women, with 91 percent of respondents over thirty years of age, with 43 percent between thirty and thirty-nine, 29 percent between forty and forty-nine, 16 percent between fifty and fifty-nine, and 3 percent over sixty. They worked for hospitals (76 percent), doctors' offices (7 percent) and surgical centers (4 percent). The remaining 13 percent were employed as sales representatives for pharmaceutical companies, were consultants, or were affiliated with university programs. There were 85 percent employed full-time; 92 percent of the respondents were Caucasian, 3 percent were African American, 3 percent were Asian, 1 percent were Hispanic, and 1 percent were Native American.

Earning power was split into four areas: 27 percent of the respondents made less than $30,000 per year, 27 percent made between $30,000 and $40,000, 21 percent made between $40,000 and $50,000, and 25 percent made over $50,000.

The respondents were highly educated, which is not unusual or surprising; working in healthcare requires education and skills. Those with RN diplomas totaled 159. In addition, 102 respondents had B.S. or B.S.N. degrees, 45 had M.A. or M.S.N. degrees, 2 had

Ph.D.s, another had an E.E.D. degree, and many were working on M.B.A. degrees. Twenty-eight of the respondents were women physicians, of whom two had begun their careers in medicine as RNs.

Job titles varied: 34 percent were directors, managers, or supervisors; 27 percent worked as RNs; 12 percent were doctors; 11 percent were in education; 7 percent worked in clerical or secretarial areas; 3 percent were technicians; 2 percent were sales representatives with pharmaceutical companies; and 4 percent worked in other areas.

One significant fact is that *percentages* of women working in the healthcare industry are significantly higher than in the general workplace. Other professional groups that contain a greater percentage of women than men include teachers, flight attendants, secretaries, paralegals, bookkeepers, bank tellers, retail workers, clerical workers, and customer service personnel. I believe that the results of my 1993 survey are indicative of those found in a female-dominated environment. The voices and personal stories do come from women working in healthcare, but their experiences and pain can be transposed to other work environments. It is also important to note that the men who participated in the 1993 survey were few in number. In two key areas—nursing and dental hygiene—women are expected to continue making up over 90 percent of their respective work forces; minimal male participation in these areas will have little impact on what women report about their working relationships with other women.

Findings

In my 1987 survey of women in the workplace, 53 percent of the women said that they had been treated unethically by another woman, and 63 percent said that they had been treated unethically by a man. The 1993 survey, based exclusively on healthcare professionals, revealed changes (see Figure 1.1). For example, 58 percent of the respondents in 1993 stated that they had been treated unethically

Figure 1.1.   Sabotage in the Workplace.

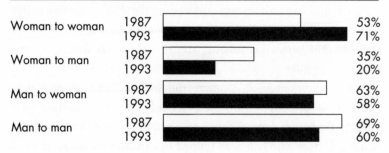

Woman to woman	1987		53%
	1993		71%
Woman to man	1987		35%
	1993		20%
Man to woman	1987		63%
	1993		58%
Man to man	1987		69%
	1993		60%

by a man at work, compared to 71 percent of the respondents who said they had been treated unethically by a woman at work. Of the male respondents, 20 percent had been treated unethically by a woman, and 60 percent had been treated unethically by a man. Within the medical field, over 75 percent of the nurses and 9 percent of the women doctors said they had been undermined by another woman. Over 80 percent of each group felt that the actions were intentional. The 1993 results illustrate a 34 percent *increase* in unethical behavior by women toward women and a 7 percent decrease of reported unethical behavior of men toward women.

In 1987, I said that men generally have more power in the workplace, and so they have more opportunities to behave unethically in the struggle to get ahead. Women are more likely to sabotage each other simply because women are more likely to work together. Women are still viewed by many as weaker in their work positioning, given their lack of experience, ignorance of the rules, naïveté, or absence from executive decision-making positions. (Granted, a small percentage of women are penetrating the "glass ceiling"; but, overall, the gains are not yet substantial enough to eliminate it.) As women move up the occupational ladder or are more likely to work with other women, they tend to encounter more unethical behavior. Why?

In addition to power and opportunity, the ramifications of fear, envy, jealousy, and low self-esteem surfaced in the 1987 interviews: if a woman (or a man) is in a titled position and has low self-esteem, it is unlikely that her or his subordinates or co-workers will be treated fairly and equally.

With the increase in women studying medicine, women now comprise 40 percent of the medical school population. In the dental field, 53 percent of dentists are women and minorities. We found that women doctors who had been trained in an authoritarian manner in medical school, internships, and residencies tended to display more verbal abuse and undermining of general work relationships. Women doctors who had been trained in or practiced participative management were far less likely to engage in verbal abuse or to undermine work relationships.

In the 1993 survey, 65 percent of the respondents said that their work relations had been undermined by unethical behavior on the part of another woman (see Figure 1.2). (The most common types of this behavior reported were verbal abuse in front of colleagues and unprofessional conduct in doctors.) This was followed by personal harassment (13 percent), discrimination (11 percent), and gossip (9 percent). Undermining of work relations was also the number one complaint about men (34 percent). Within that grouping, 43 percent of the respondents said they had been verbally abused, and 23 percent said they had been sexually harassed (the respondents separated derogatory remarks from verbal abuse, but most derogatory comments contained sexual innuendo).

Only 11 percent stated that they felt sabotage by a man was not intentional (see Figure 1.3); 84 percent stated that it was definitely intentional, and 5 percent were not sure. Only 7 percent of the respondents felt that unethical treatment by a woman was not intentional; 84 percent said it was definitely intentional, and 7 percent were not sure.

The question arises of why women would purposely undermine

Fig

Cau

Figure 1.2. Causes of Sabotaging Behavior.

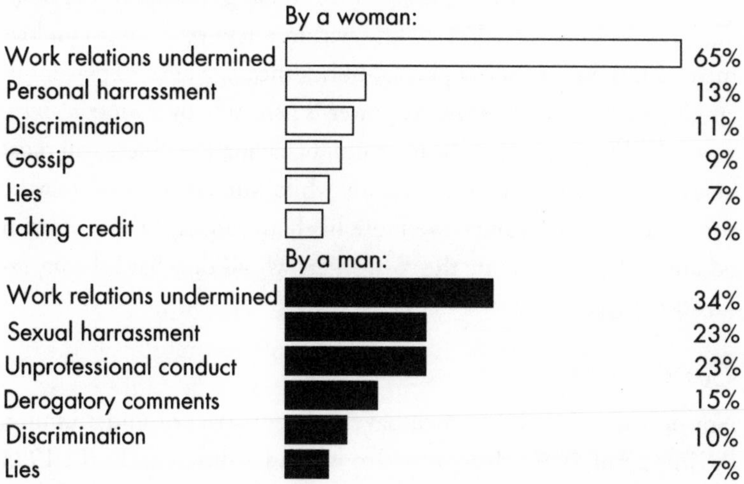

By a woman:

Work relations undermined	65%
Personal harrassment	13%
Discrimination	11%
Gossip	9%
Lies	7%
Taking credit	6%

By a man:

Work relations undermined	34%
Sexual harrassment	23%
Unprofessional conduct	23%
Derogatory comments	15%
Discrimination	10%
Lies	7%

and sabotage other women in an environment that is supposed to reflect nurturing, caring, and getting well. Do nurses "eat their young," as many women said in the follow-up interviews?

Women and Men: Differences

Both the 1987 and 1993 surveys indicated that women are more likely to behave unethically toward women than they are toward men.

Figure 1.3. Intentionality.

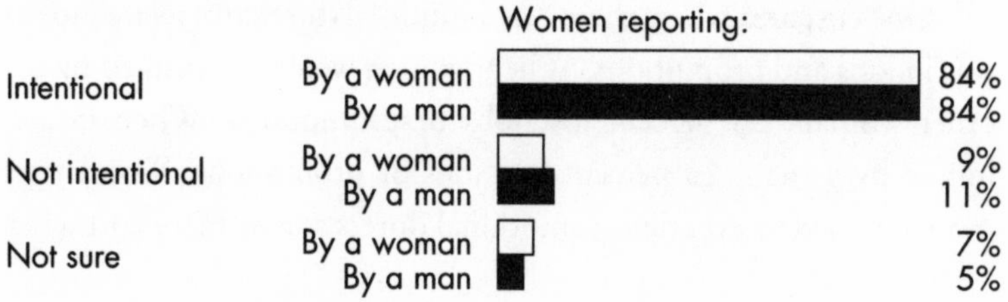

Women reporting:

Intentional	By a woman	84%
	By a man	84%
Not intentional	By a woman	9%
	By a man	11%
Not sure	By a woman	7%
	By a man	5%

Why? In healthcare, men usually run things. Women may rise to a specific level (such as vice president for nursing) but then they stop. Staff nurses hit their salary ceiling within a few years after employment. Thus, in the "velvet ghetto" of healthcare, where 70 percent of employees are female, women's power is generally over *other women*, and so if there is going to be unethical behavior, the object will most likely be another woman. Therefore, while women and men may be equally unethical, women are more likely to sabotage other women because other women are the co-workers whom they have the *opportunity* to undermine.

Costs

Not only do men and women have different styles of undermining, the impact of their behavior toward women is different. In the 1993 study, women reported that when they had been undermined by anyone, a man or a woman, the primary cost was embarrassment (see Figure 1.4). But 61 percent of the women reported such embarrassment when they had been undermined by another woman, while 74 percent reported embarrassment after having been undermined by a man. This discrepancy may be due to the male-female roles that society dictates. A woman may be more likely to feel that she must have done something to cause the other person to undermine her, particularly if the person has a higher status than she does. In most cases, the person with higher status, such as a physician, is a man. But when she is undermined by another woman, she will feel that they are on more equal footing; her reaction is more likely to include anger.

One cost area where there was a minimal difference related to sex was in jobs and promotions. When women were undermined by another woman, 25 percent lost jobs or promotions. When undermined by a man, 23 percent lost jobs or promotions. Women are more inclined to experience emotional duress as a primary cost when

Figure 1.4. Cost Factors.

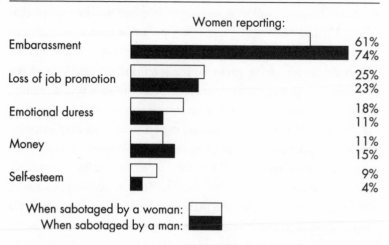

	Women reporting:
Embarassment	61% / 74%
Loss of job promotion	25% / 23%
Emotional duress	18% / 11%
Money	11% / 15%
Self-esteem	9% / 4%

When sabotaged by a woman:
When sabotaged by a man:

undermined by a woman (18 percent) than when undermined by a man (11 percent).

Money was also a factor: 11 percent of the women respondents stated that they had lost money because of undermining by other women. The primary cause was embezzlement; several of the women physicians stated that many thousands of dollars had been stolen by female employees. The primary cost of undermining by men was money for 15 percent of the respondents.

Women also reported that their self-esteem had been reduced or shattered more when another woman undermined them (9 percent) than when a man sabotaged them (4 percent). My 1987 study showed that men tend to be more pragmatically oriented when they decided to do someone in: the reason for sabotage is usually money or someone else's job. The same study found that women tend to react more personally or emotionally to sabotage than men do.

Many of the women who reported having experienced a financial disaster or loss of a job also reported secondary factors that surfaced later on. Women employers seemed to fare better. They stated that when the undermining behavior was performed by a woman employee, the primary cost was embarrassment, followed by low morale. When the undermining came from a man, the primary cost to the employer was perceived by women to be nothing; it was as though when a man undermined a woman, it was acceptable—no big deal.

Does society (or the workplace) expect men to display inappropriate, unsupportive, undermining behavior? Women's responses indicated that this may be so. Therefore, there may be less severe reactions or responses to inappropriate behavior by men: it comes with the territory. In healthcare, the majority of practicing doctors are still men, and most hospitals subscribe to the premise that they are in the business of supporting doctors' needs.

When one person sabotages another, the saboteur seeks to gain something, while the sabotaged person may lose something. In the 1993 survey, 40 percent of the respondents said that when they were undermined by another woman, she intended to enhance her own reputation; 19 percent said she intended to gain power; and 12 percent declared that either a promotion or job was the saboteur's goal (see Figure 1.5). When the saboteur was a man, 23 percent of the respondents said that enhanced reputation was his goal, and 13 percent said it was additional power. Very few reported men gaining jobs or promotions through sabotage. In healthcare, as in business, men already occupy most positions of authority; they may not see any other gains but enhanced reputations or visibility.

"Nothing" was the answer that 17 percent of the respondents gave when asked what an employer gained by a woman's unethical behavior. If an employer were to gain anything from a man's unethical behavior, 5 percent of the respondents stated, it would be the employer's enhanced reputation or visibility; otherwise, the majority of respondents said, employers gained nothing when men undermined

Figure 1.5. Gains from Sabotage.

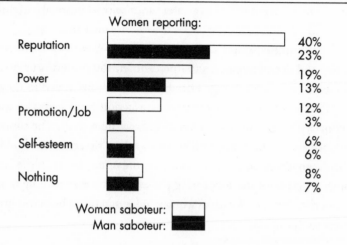

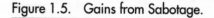

them. Losses to the employer were another matter. Whether the saboteurs were men or women, loss of reputation, of employees' loyalty,
of employees' productivity, of credibility, of team growth, and of effectiveness were all factors.

Different Visions

Men and women come to the workplace with dissimilar rules and
motivations that affect how they act and dictate what is important.
Usually, for men, the main focus is on bottom-line factors: success in
material terms, doing a job or task for money. Historically, women's
work was often a stopgap measure, or simply something to do.
Money is now a factor for women, of course, but there are others: reputation, visibility, and self-esteem all rank high.

In healthcare, people can be viewed as players on a field. The
main players are key hospital administrators and doctors. The doctors do most of the "scoring." Their focus is on what the score is (how
many patients, how much revenue generated), how to increase the

score for themselves (higher fees, bigger payouts), and how to keep others from making gains (greater clout within hospitals' exclusive specialties).

The spectators and supporting players—nurses (97 percent female) and dental hygienists (99 percent female)—don't usually have the same focus on scoring. They become more interested in tangential things. The main players gain satisfaction from seeing or interacting with other spectators (the "old boys' network"). The supporting players are interested in being noticed, so that they can build up their own reputations and be chosen more often to play in the game. Since so many of the supporting players are women, making money is not their primary focus, as women are less likely to be in important executive positions.

Saboteurs

One question that arises is whether a female saboteur would purposely target another woman. In the 1993 survey, I asked whether the saboteur's action had anything to do with the respondent's being a woman or a man. I found 52 percent who said yes—that the action directed against them by a woman was a direct reflection of their gender; 38 percent said no, and 10 percent were not sure. I found 76 percent who stated that a man had sabotaged them because of their sex; 20 percent said men had not, and 4 percent were not sure.

In the 1987 study, I found a big difference of opinion between most men and women on this point. Most of the women in the original survey believed that when a man treated them unethically, he was taking advantage of them because they were women; many of the women accused the men of sexism and sexual harassment. Men didn't think that their sex had anything to do with being sabotaged; they believed that those who acted unethically toward them did so because of other reasons.

The Gender of Choice

Unethical behavior by women, as reported in the 1987 survey, was believed to have a gender-related component by male and female respondents alike. In 1987, 60 percent of the previous respondents thought there was a relationship between what had happened and their own gender; 62 percent of the women and 48 percent of the men felt that there was such a relationship involved in unethical treatment by a woman; 80 percent of the women and 15 percent of the men felt there was such a relationship in unethical treatment by a man.

In the 1993 survey, 59 percent of the women felt that there was a gender-based relationship when unethical treatment came from a woman, and 76 percent said there was when it came from a man (see Figure 1.6). Although the present study indicates a decline in this perception about women, there is a footnote. In subsequent interviews with 100 of the 227 respondents, several (11) who had indicated no such relationship on the survey changed their minds during the in-

Figure 1.6.   Gender as a Factor in Being Sabotaged.

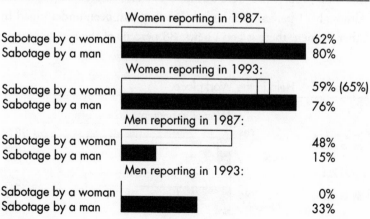

Women reporting in 1987:	
Sabotage by a woman	62%
Sabotage by a man	80%
Women reporting in 1993:	
Sabotage by a woman	59% (65%)
Sabotage by a man	76%
Men reporting in 1987:	
Sabotage by a woman	48%
Sabotage by a man	15%
Men reporting in 1993:	
Sabotage by a woman	0%
Sabotage by a man	33%

terviews. This change would increase, from 59 percent to 65 percent, the number saying that being a woman is a factor in sabotage by another woman.

A substantial number of the women felt that women's undermining other women comes with the territory. Since the majority of employees in their workplaces were women, it was assumed that there would be undermining, and that it would be directed at them.

As mentioned earlier, the men in the study were very few: 5 out of 227. Of the male respondents, 4 out of 5 stated they had been treated unethically, 3 by a man and 1 by a woman. Only 1 felt that his treatment was a reflection of his gender. There may be a connection here with intentionality; see Figure 1.3.

Support and Lack of Support

There are always two sides to every coin. The flip side of not supporting someone is helping someone in the workplace. In the study, I looked for connections between who supports and who doesn't support another. Those who usually have the power to help also have the power to behave unethically. In the interviews, it often appeared that the same people who were unsupportive also offered help at times. Although 71 percent responded that they had been undermined by other women, there is good news: 88 percent of the survey respon-

Figure 1.7.   Help in the Workplace.

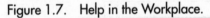

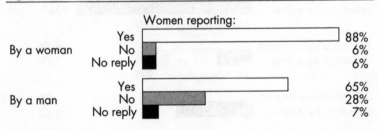

Figure 1.8.   Gender as a Factor in Help.

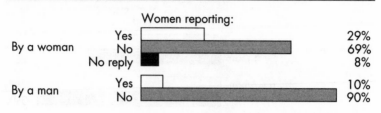

dents had been actively helped by a woman, and 65 percent had been actively helped by a man. With a greater female population in the healthcare field, it's logical that more women would report being helped as well as harmed by other women (see Figure 1.7).

When we asked if gender had anything to do with the amount of help received, 69 percent said it did not when the help came from women, and 90 percent said their gender had nothing to do with help from a male (see Figure 1.8).

When women were helped by other women, 34 percent stated that they had been supported, 28 percent stated that a woman was very helpful, 14 percent said women were mentors, and 12 percent said that women had involved them in teamwork. Men had been very helpful to 39 percent of the respondents; 28 percent found men supportive, 10 percent were mentored, and 7 percent were included by men in teamwork (see Figure 1.9). Finally, when it came to receiving assistance in getting a job or a promotion, women stated that they were more likely to get help from other women.

Preference

Since healthcare is predominantly women working together, some might assume that women would choose to work in healthcare because of that factor. Our respondents stated that they do choose to work with women (30 percent), or that they have no preference for

Figure 1.9.   Descriptions of Help in the Workplace.

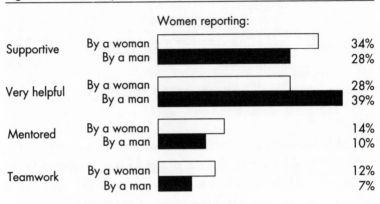

working with either sex (36 percent). An alarming 34 percent stated that they preferred not to work with women (see Figure 1.10). Women said they did not care to work with women because women are untrustworthy, backbiting, backstabbing, covert, gossipy, unsure of themselves, and unbusinesslike. The reasons they gave for preferring to work with men were that men are more straightforward, businesslike, job-oriented, and clearer about what the rules are.

Giving and Getting

There was a connection between helpfulness and preferences. Those who had a gender preference were more likely to find that the pre-

Figure 1.10.   Gender Preferences.

Women reporting:	
Prefer to work with women	30%
Prefer to work with men	34%
Either	36%

ferred gender was more helpful than those who had no such preference. It's important to note that some of the reasons given for preferences do reflect traditional stereotypes about how women behave, as well as the styles of unethical behavior discussed earlier. Respondents who prefer to work with women may have a personal bias toward women or feel they need support from other women.

Those respondents who expressed a preference for working with men stated they believed men were less petty, less likely to play games, or less likely to have personal or emotional problems (no one in the returned surveys referred to premenstrual syndrome or menopause). They also tended to say that women who act unethically and undermine others do so by being deceptive, vindictive, and covert.

Friendships

The questionnaire for the 1993 survey asked the respondents if they had developed friendships at work, and 70 percent said yes (see Figure 1.11). Reasons given by those who said no included needing to be more careful, needing more time time to develop friendships, preferring only professional relationships with co-workers, thinking friendships should be avoided with employees, and being shy, selective, or too busy.

Respondents were also asked whether they regretted having befriended a woman or a man at work. I found that 45 percent regret-

Figure 1.11. Friendships at Work.

		Women reporting:	
Developed friendships quickly at work	Yes		70%
	No		23%
	No response		7%

Figure 1.12.   Regret About Friendships at Work.

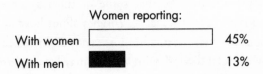

ted befriending a woman, and 13 percent regretted befriending a man (see Figure 1.12). Reasons given for regretting friendships with women included misuse of personal information, being stabbed in the back, false friendship, manipulation, and getting too personal (see Figure 1.13). With men, the reasons included sexual harassment, personal harassment, dishonesty, and being manipulated. One woman psychiatrist said that she had befriended a woman, invited her home, and introduced her to her family. The new "friend" ended up having an affair with her husband, which led to a divorce. Having

Figure 1.13.   Reasons for Regretting Friendships.

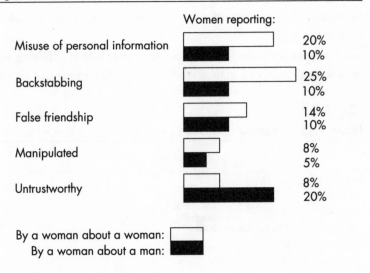

a friend pursue my spouse would fit my definition of unethical behavior.

Et Tu?

The last question on the 1993 survey asked was "Have you ever been accused of unethical behavior?" There were 10 percent who said yes, 82 percent who said no, and 8 percent who weren't sure (see Figure 1.14). Of those who said yes, most said the reason was unprofessional behavior. Other reasons were being a poor loser, having one's actions misunderstood, using improper procedures, creating work-related conflicts, and lying. All the respondents who reported having been accused of unethical behavior also reported that they had been treated unethically by others. My previous research had shown that the more a person experienced unethical behavior from others, the more that person was likely to be accused of the same things, justifiably or not.

In the 1987 study, men were twice as likely as women to be accused of unethical behavior. Moreover, 38 percent of the men who reported unethical treatment by both men and women claimed that they had been accused themselves, whereas only 20 percent of the women admitted to any accusations. That difference could be telling: if there were more men working in healthcare, I suspect that the respondents from the 1993 study would parallel the 1987 study in this area.

Figure 1.14.   Being Accused of Unethical Behavior.

	Women reporting:	
Yes		10%
No		82%
Not sure		8%

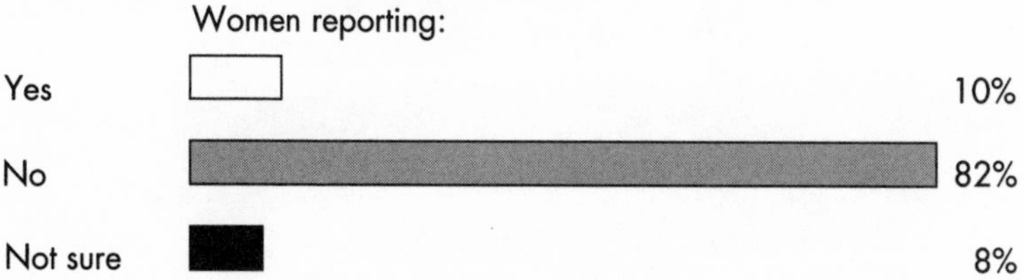

The 1987 study suggests that men may be better able to strike back, and do strike back (or others perceive that they do). In contrast, women who are less powerful are often less likely to be accused of action directed at men, since there are fewer men at their level. Others are less likely to perceive women as aggressors. If a woman is going to be an aggressor, she will direct her attention at an individual who she believes or perceives to have less power in the workplace—another woman.

The bottom line is that it's a power game. Unfortunately, our culture translates success into dollars, and unethical behavior becomes part of it. To change unethical and sabotaging behavior, we must come to terms with power issues. Their dynamics need to be investigated and explored. Finally, a method of dealing with power needs to be established in ways that will be beneficial to both women and men in the healthcare field.

Both sexes behave unethically, although their styles and methods are different. But sabotaging behavior is not genetic. It is learned, and it can be unlearned.

2

Why Women Undermine
Other Women

Healthcare is synonymous with caring and nurturing. Why was there a greater reporting of women's undermining women in my 1993 study of women in healthcare than in the 1987 study of women in the general workplace? This chapter tells why women undermine other women, and why there has been an increase in reports of women's sabotaging behavior.

The Problem

The problem is twofold: women working with women, and women not wanting to work with women. Our 1993 study indicated that one-third of the women respondents did not want to work with or for another woman, whereas two-thirds of the respondents had no objection. Since 70 percent of healthcare employees are women, a potentially dangerous environment for both patients and working personnel occurs.

Women traditionally have been drawn to the healthcare field, and their percentages are expected to increase during the next decade. Today, women are still society's caregivers. The pay is reasonable, with 70 percent of all the respondents from my study indicating they made in excess of $30,000 and one-quarter of all respondents making in excess of $50,000.

Dialogue with the various segments within healthcare points to a widespread fear of the unknown. Its members don't know where the industry is going with the reforms, much less where it will take them. This could prove to be a classic situation: the survival of the fittest, with battles being fought by both overt and subtle manipulations. Many players will be rendered obsolete, some will come away dismayed and distressed, and others will look at it as an opportunity to grow and expand in whatever they are now doing. In addition to fear of the unknown, demographics, history, psychology, and sociology reveal eleven major reasons why women are inclined to undermine their own sex:

1. There is greater competition among women within the workplace today. This is due to both demographic and social trends. Women struggle harder to obtain their positions and get ahead, many being the primary source of income for their homes.

2. The downturn of the economy during the 1990s has pitted woman against woman when it comes to layoffs. As a rule, women are not in senior management; they are employed in middle to lower management, if in management at all. When layoffs and terminations are presented, women are often the first to go.

3. Present-day society is continuing to experience crises of unethical behavior. Traditional morals and values have declined. The impact seems to be greater on women; they have traditionally held the family together (however the family is defined), setting the tone for its values, its ethics, and its morals.

4. The workplace is still a jungle, with the players struggling to take advantage of various opportunities and to form alliances. The biggest change to affect the healthcare industry in the 1990s will be the reform proposed by the Clinton administration.

5. Women are known to be practitioners of a participative management style. Their personal style works successfully at times. At other times, it can backfire because of its greater personal interaction with colleagues and employees.

6. If discipline, a reprimand, or criticism are warranted in a specific situation, one may feel betrayed because there was a perceived personal relationship with the supervisor. This is far more common with women than with men. Women are more likely to develop personal relationships with other women in the workplace. Men don't view personal relationships as a priority.

7. Women are overloaded. They have extra pressures from balancing their family and workplace responsibilities, as well as their personal lives. Jane and Robert Handley, authors of *Why Women Worry,* state that because women are overloaded, attempting to balance work with family and personal life, they worry more. Their worries cover relationships, appearance, pleasing, making wrong decisions, health, kids, lack of time, aging, parents, job performance, and even world affairs. Men are much more myopic in their concerns.

8. Women are still held back from upper-level management positions because of old stereotypes. A woman still has to do and accomplish more before she is viewed as someone of competence. In healthcare, over 2 million women hold

97 percent of nursing positions. Nurses quickly hit the "glass ceiling." Their ability to advance, as well as to enhance their income, is severely limited.

9. Upbringing is always a factor. Women have been raised differently from men, and they bring a more flexible and situational approach to relating the world to the workplace. Those approaches and methods are consistently passed on to the next generation.

10. Women and men are split on their psychological realities. Each sex relates to the world differently, and so each has different ideas about dishonesty and deception, competition, self-esteem, and the impact of relationships. Men deal differently with their feelings of anger and hostility.

11. Women are acknowledging that they have been undermined by other women. In the past, women ignored it, didn't talk about it, or denied that another woman had displayed sabotaging behavior toward them or others. If a woman spoke up and spoke out, she could be misinterpreted as not supporting other women.

Denial Is In

With my publication of *Woman to Woman*, in 1987, many women's groups and associations were angry that I had pointed out the fact of these differences. They suggested that women in the workplace should be viewed as the equals of men, and they believed that any discussion about differences or disparities would only hurt women in the end.

To deny these differences is absurd. There is no question that women should have equal opportunity, and that women have the ability to do virtually any job on the same level as their male counterparts. That is a separate issue, however. The issue that I am addressing is the fact that women don't support other women. This appears to permeate female-dominated professions, such as nursing, dentistry, teaching, secretarial services, and the cosmetology industry.

What we see, then, are differences that women bring to the workplace and how these can interfere with women working together. The workplace can change. Women can become more aware of what is happening and conscientiously control any destructive behavior that erupts. Through our shared knowledge of awareness, confronting, and speaking out, women will learn to support each other more effectively.

Social Trends

Demographics and social trends are major factors in the status of women in the workplace. The past two decades have seen a rapid overall transformation in the workplace. Women have moved in growing numbers into higher-level positions. Their employment has been a key factor in the shift toward services and away from manufacturing and industry.

Parity in the paycheck has not yet occurred. In 1980, women earned only 60 percent of what men earned. In 1984, the average increased to 64 percent; in 1990, to 70 percent. It is estimated that by the year 2000, women will be earning at least 74 percent of what men earn.[1] Women are continually getting more education, experience, and recognition and are moving into higher-level jobs. As women perform well in their new jobs, doors will continue to open. Recent statistics support this prediction.

Women Working in Health Care

Since 1970, the number of women in management and professional jobs has escalated; women are moving into professions formerly dominated by men. During the 1970s, women held only 18 percent of executive, administrative, and management positions. By 1980, they held 30 percent.[2] Employment in the healthcare field grew by more than 2.5 million jobs in the 1980s, to 7.8 million in 1990. It is estimated that by the year 2005, 11.5 million women and men will be employed in this field.

Registered nurses (RNs) compose the largest segment of employment in healthcare. The U.S. Department of Labor projects that the number will reach 2,018,000 by the year 2000. Present estimates from various nursing associations estimate the number to exceed 2.5 million. However, the data on current training include the startling estimate that by the year 2000 there will be only half the number of nurses needed.[3]

The particular need for increased nursing personnel is largely a function of the AIDS epidemic, which is having and will continue to have a profound effect on the entire healthcare industry. The majority of people reported to have AIDS are between the ages of twenty and forty-five. The number of AIDS cases among women and infants continues to grow. It is projected that the impact of the AIDS epidemic will accelerate over the next few years, until a cure is found. Many believe that predictions of a nurse shortage by the year 2000 is underestimated.[4]

The demand for RNs continues to rise, but the supply decreases. In the fall of 1986, 20,000 female college freshmen planned to become nurses, compared to 43,000 in 1983. The University of California at Los Angeles reported a 50 percent decrease since 1974 of women interested in pursuing a nursing career, as opposed to an almost threefold increase among those interested in business.

In 1984, 8.3 percent of female college freshmen were aspiring nurses. By 1986, the number had decreased to 5.1 percent. Today, many women are choosing to become physicians instead of nurses, because they now have this option. In 1991, American colleges awarded 14,500 bachelor of science in nursing (B.S.N.) degrees, compared to almost 16,000 medical degrees to women. The last numbers are eye-opening. They place the much-discussed physician surplus and nursing shortage in an interesting and very different light.[5] In 1992 and 1993, many hospitals created hiring freezes, even though there was a definite need and positions were available. Few were being filled because of the uncertainty of healthcare reform.

Many women work because they have to. They are heads of households, or their earnings are needed in two-income families. The social changes that propelled women into the work force have created other pressures. Divorce rates have increased, and more women choose to remain single.

Women are gaining more responsibility in the workplace, but they also have more responsibilities outside the workplace. Women have more freedom and choice in their lives, but freedom and choice also bring risk.

Women have increased financial responsibility for themselves and their families. This is enhanced by the increase in divorce rates and is statistically supported by the fact that a great majority of women who are awarded child or spousal support do not actually receive it. They become financially overburdened because of these non-payments. Many women feel alone. When they concentrate on their work, careers, or family, especially if they are heads of households, they often don't have the time or the energy to develop other relationships.

The ongoing income gap between men and women adds pressure. Women are often trapped into lower-paying, routine jobs in the "pink-collar ghetto." In 1982, 99 percent of all secretaries were women.[6] In 1994, 99 percent of all secretaries are still women. Granted, there are women who will break away from the pack; but when they do, it often becomes a source of resentment and hurt to those left behind.

Outcasts from Within

Many of the women I interviewed in 1993 and 1987 reported that when they received promotions, they often found themselves in an "out group" environment. No longer were they in the inner circle, privy to shared confidences or even what would be construed as "girlfriend chat." They were now considered outcasts: women who had broken out were not to be trusted.

Pressures also occur with women who are outside a big corporation. According to recent statistics, women-owned businesses employ more individuals nationwide than the *Fortune* 500 companies combined. Women started their own businesses at a ratio of three to one over men throughout the 1980s. The 1990s are projected to be no different. For many women, leaving a company and starting a business is a direct response to some form of corporate discrimination. They often feel blocked from advancement, and so their only way out is to do their own thing.

Once in business for themselves, however, women face more pressures. Since men have been creating businesses for a long time, women now run smack into the "old boys' network" and the new "old boys' network"—the next generation. As more and more women jump into the entrepreneurial mode and start their own businesses, they are developing their own support networks. In Denver, for example, there are over thirty professional women's groups that offer networking support under the Colorado Women's Leadership Coalition.

Like these businesswomen, many nurses have broken away from a traditional employee-employer relationship with hospitals and formed their own co-ops, negotiating directly with hospitals for their services. Within their co-ops, they have associates and junior and senior partners. These entrepreneurial nurses have found that they are more in control of their own destinies and their own dollars.

Because women gravitate toward the service types of businesses, their competitors are usually going to be other women, especially in the beginning stages. Therefore, they are more likely to direct their competitive actions toward other women than toward men, who have been out there longer, are more established, and are more entrenched in the corporate environment.

Stereotype Overload

Women are still burdened with expectations and stereotypes of what they should do and how they should behave. These stereotypes specify that women should do certain types of work. They should emphasize their nurturing skills and their domestic abilities, as well as their physical attractiveness. Women are brought up to believe that they should be friends with everybody, and that friends don't usually compete with other friends But it is naïve to assume that everyone will be a friend or should be; the reality is that not everyone is friend material. When a woman opens up too soon about her hopes and dreams, her fears and concerns, she may be opening up to the wrong person. That person, usually another woman, may use this newly gained information against her. A woman who is open, in the spirit of girlhood-inspired niceness, may come to feel personally betrayed.

Men learn something different. They are taught as boys to concentrate and to expand their technical skills and physical abilities, as well as to be domineering and authoritative.

Old habits, patterns and attitudes die hard. Today's women play a different and newer role in the workplace as they break from the old stereotypes of being supporters and caregivers. Many people, men as well as women, feel uncomfortable with the role changes.

In the mid 1980s, the *Wall Street Journal* published a survey in which 29 percent of the women said that they would rather work for men because they believed female executives were too petty and too critical. They felt that their female bosses were overcompensating by being overbearing. The feeling was that because female bosses had to work so hard to succeed, they demanded much more of their subordinates. The participants in the survey also felt that some of their female bosses were too easily threatened, and that they perceived their positions as being in jeopardy. Since there were relatively fewer opportunities for women executives, the ones who succeeded were more competitive.[7]

In June 1993, *Working Woman* magazine released its reader-survey results on women bosses: 23 percent of the participants stated that they preferred a male boss.[8] My 1993 study found 34 percent of respondents who preferred not working with other women.

The women's movement has definitely been a force in creating new roles, perceptions, and realities for women in the workplace. It also helped create the present situation, which contributes to women's undermining of other women. My survey revealed that when women are under a great deal of stress, they are far more likely to sabotage each other, since they have to compete for a finite number of positions. At the same time, women's vulnerability opens up. These factors all contribute to women's sabotaging each other.

Women and the Decline of Values

The war on values and the decline of values is broadcast daily in the newspapers, on television, and on the radio. Examples are everywhere: religious disputes, drugs, guns, and ethical debates over developments in science and medicine. The movie *Jurassic Park* stimulated a debate on whether science should leave well enough alone. Apathy seems to be everywhere. Many people just don't care, or they feel that if they are not directly involved in a situation, it is not their problem. In an article published in *Fortune* magazine almost twenty years ago, Peter Berger traces how religious education and scientific institutions have been hit hard by ethical decline. One of his main points is that the values of the secular and the religious cultures alike in America have been undermined and weakened. Even as they claim to support these values, people have lost faith in traditions and institutions.[9]

The impact on women is substantial. Historically, they have been constrained by traditional values. As values change, so do the constraints on women. People become confused about what to do when beliefs about what is proper break down.

Individuals may have one standard of ethics, and the company they work for may have another. The employees jointly may have a group ethic that is different from the ethics of the separate individuals as well as from the ethic of the company. Thomas J. Hayes describes this when he says, "The employee's dilemma is compounded when he or she seeks out a single moral standard to follow and one does not exist."[10]

Many businesses and hospitals actually create an environment that can contribute to unethical actions. Multiple departments lead to conflicting institutional goals, or there may be a disparity between short-term and long-term profit goals. If problems arise in one unit of an organization, some within the unit may seek to shift the blame to another unit.

In interviews with one hundred women and men for this book, several respondents cited examples from their own organizations, where cutbacks and layoffs were routinely in effect but management continued to enjoy condominium privileges, country clubs, use of company cars, and even clothing allowances. These were items and perks that most employees did not enjoy during good times, much less in bad times. In the 1970s, David Linowes gave a speech on international business and morality. His speech is as appropriate today as it was then. In it, he said, "Our environment suffers from confusion as to what is morally right and wrong. The danger is serious, because immorality and dishonesty are contagious. They spread and grow when left in their own condoning environment"[11]

This pervasive breakdown of values is nothing new. Vast technological and social changes have disrupted traditional roles and relationships. As society has let down its hair and as morals and values have loosened, everyone is freer to act on his or her own "druthers." No one is immune to these social changes, including women. Their position in society has changed the most over the past two decades, and they may be more at risk because of their own roles and relationships.

Social and Cultural Dynamics in the Workplace

Are there competitive pressures in the workplace that are especially stressful to women? Are there special circumstances that make women even more likely to undermine other women, or is it just office politics?

The Corporate Barrier

Working Woman magazine annually features the top one hundred companies that are the best ones for women to work for. The baby boomers are getting older. With children, they have child-care needs as well as elder-care needs. Corporations today appear to be more humane, offering a variety of family-related services.

But most large corporations are highly complex, with many levels of power, and power encourages a variety of coalitions and factions to form. These groups serve two purposes: they provide a source of strength and nurturing, and they offer a power base for people working their way to the top. As individuals move from one group to another, they can easily step on others. The ones stepped on become hostile and resentful.

Thus one of the results of a more altruistic environment is that pathways and communication routes to top management are more open, and individual creativity is encouraged. And there are more opportunities for employees to develop power groups, factions, and coalitions to achieve their personal goals. A consequence is that women are more apt to be exploited or to prey on other women in the ensuing power struggles. Why? When a woman preys on or stalks someone else, the target will usually be someone with less power— most likely another woman.

In *Corporate Cultures*, Deal and Kennedy identify the obstacles that make it hard for women to merge into a corporate culture. The majority of corporate women they interviewed felt excluded from important events at many stages in their careers. The men already in power tended not to see them. The first edition of the book was published in 1982. Its reflection of the early 1980s is similar to what goes on in the 1990s, especially in large companies.

Women commonly react to such barriers by feeling frustrated and powerless. It's difficult to act out their hostile feelings toward those in power—the men. That leaves the less powerful—women— as the targets. Women know these barriers are in place and may struggle even harder to get into the inner, more powerful circles. If it means they have to push other women down to get there, that's the breaks.

Underground Players

Subcultures spring up in companies for a variety of reasons. Most likely, they develop around work differences. Examples are groups centered on sales, research and development, dentistry, critical-care nursing, and surgery. They also develop around common economic, educational, and gender characteristics. Once formed, groups create their own cultural environments and world views. Anyone with low power in these groups feels disappointed when her own values and opinions are not recognized. She in turn penalizes those who have even less power, and the pecking order goes into effect.

Secretaries and clerks are examples. As Rosabeth Moss Kanter found in studying men and women in corporations, secretaries sometimes got caught up in power struggles. She learned that each secretary's status was linked to that of her boss. The secretaries of the higher-level bosses would dump on the secretaries of the lower-level bosses when they saw their bosses feuding. (Sometimes they even undermined their own bosses when they had designs on the bosses' jobs. This scenario was likely to occur when the boss was a woman, since the position seemed more attainable if it was already held by another woman.) In healthcare, this commonly happens in male doctor–female nurse relationships. A nurse may identify her power with that of her employer, the chief of staff, or even the doctor who generates the most revenues for the hospital.

As women move up the corporate ladder, ideal conditions for sabotaging behavior can flourish. Kanter noticed that some individuals would gain the advantage of being fast-tracked as prime officer candidates. They had more career reviews, and they were moved into positions where they were more likely to become targets of resentment for those not so favored. Meanwhile, many of their peers suddenly warmed up to them, in order to be part of a winner's team.[12]

Getting ahead requires skills, including the skill of maneuvering through the resentment of those left behind. Getting ahead is like a game. Doing it is important, and therefore it is stressed for both women and men. But women have fewer resources and fewer skills for playing the game than men do. Until they learn the rules, they may be more likely to engage in questionable conduct against each other.

Another problem surfaces: since there are fewer women at the higher corporate levels, women in these positions are more visible.

Some may view women's behavior on the way to the top as tricky or devious. It can be a no-win situation if they want to survive in the business world. The game is now harder and has more constraints. Women haven't learned all the rules, nor have they passed them on to other women when they have learned them. Their actions can be construed as more calculating than men's. In the end, women are more likely to be accused of foul play.

Politics at Work

Political game playing can also result in women's resorting to more covert tactics. It is still not as acceptable for women as it is for men to exercise blatant power. Women aren't as open and aggressive about wanting to get to the top as men are, and so they are more likely to engage in behind-the-scenes actions. If covert methods don't work and they find themselves blocked, feelings of hostility can arise out of disappointments. As Kanter remarks, "Previous research has found that high-mobility situations tend to fester rivalry, instability in the composition of work groups, [and] comparison upward in the hierarchy."[13] Since women are more likely to be in this type of situation than men are when they try to advance, they may be more likely to express hostility and anger.

Women who choose not to aspire higher are not necessarily more ethical than those who do. According to research, including Kanter's, these women also may be deceptive, sometimes even malicious and vengeful. When they exhibit these tendencies, they often pick on people outside the group, as a way of fortifying their own low aspirations and group bonding. If someone within the group decides to promote herself and aspire higher by leaving the group, she may end up being ostracized by the others, who then assert the values and power of the group. Joking, ridicule, and taking credit for the accomplishments of the resented outsider are normal responses. Both of my studies affirm these postures.

Women are not the only practitioners of this type of behavior. Men in low-status positions may be deceptive, too, but people who act this way are more typically women. As Kanter found, women are usually in the low-status, blocked jobs, and their victims are most likely the women who have moved up the ladder. Finding fewer and fewer female peers and supporters on the way up, they are most susceptible to an assault. As men move up, they find peer groups at every level.[14]

The opposite also happens: those who move up sometimes sabotage those left behind in the trenches. It's a method of gaining revenge for past resentments and hostilities, or of affirming connections with the new group.[15] An example would be a woman who has been promoted and gives negative references for women who helped move her along.

Women as Bosses

The study published in the June 1993 issue of *Working Woman*, on women bosses, reflected 2,250 responses. Queried about placement within their organizations, the respondents stated that 49 percent of middle-management positions were held by males and 27 percent by females; 19 percent stated that there was equal representation of both sexes in middle management. As would be expected, the respondents said that 75 percent of top management was male and 9 percent female, with the remaining 16 percent split between the sexes. Only 12 percent of the respondents were in top management; 32 percent were in middle management, and 23 percent were in lower management. The remaining respondents were spread between nonsupervisory professional or specialist positions, at 18 percent; clerical worker and administrative assistant positions, at 11 percent; and service worker, at 4 percent.[16] When women are in a routine low-power setting, where the majority of women are still found, they are likely to engage in covert political activities.

The Bees

The Queen Bee is well known in the workplace. She is the woman at the top who got there by hard work. She will claim her position is due to her efforts and hers alone. Her attitude is one of nonmentoring and nonsupport of other women. She is extremely territorial and feels that any woman who wants to advance has to do it the hard way—just as she did, with no help.

In the 1980s, she was joined by the Princess Bee, who is supportive of other women within her own work environment—that is, as long as the other women do not invade her territory, her hive. In a hospital, if she is in marketing and another woman is in education, she will actively support the other woman as long as the latter shows no desire to move into marketing. The Princess Bee openly supports women moving up. She is an active mentor of other women, as long as she believes that her job and her future work are nonclaimable.

The 1990s introduced the next generation, the Phantom Bee. She is a woman who, when asked if she knows of any women who are qualified to fill a position that she is about to vacate, says: "There is no one. There is not another woman who can do the job as well as I do. I will keep my eyes open and let you know when I have found a woman who is qualified." The result is that a man often gets the promotion, and the pipeline for bringing women to the top narrows.

What's disturbing about the Bees is the shift in attitudes among younger managers. In the *Working Woman* survey, 61 percent of women forty and older believed that women have a responsibility to help other women climb the corporate ladder. Only 45 percent of those under thirty supported that philosophy.[17] This could mean that newer, younger managers may be closing the pipeline before other competent and qualified women have an opportunity.

In addition, 83 percent of the respondents said that the best way to help women is to mentor them and set a good example. Overall, 34 percent of the respondents stated that women bosses were tougher on female employees, and 30 percent preferred working for a male boss.

Respondents who earned under $15,000 per year reported greater dissatisfaction with female bosses; 47 percent of this group reported that women bosses are harder on women, compared to only 20 percent of women earning over $75,000 dollars per year.

According to 54 percent of the *Working Woman* respondents, female managers have a special responsibility to help other women rise through the ranks, and 69 percent felt that women bosses should advocate family- and female-friendly personnel policies. Over half of the women earning over $75,000 stated that they mentor as many men as they do women, and 34 percent of them stated that they do not view themselves as different from male managers.[18]

Some individuals use their connections with an advocate higher up to undercut a boss whose position ranks lower. As a strategy, a woman may act to ensure her own power base by making alliances with more than one mentor. Then, if one sponsor falls, she won't go down with the ship. This hedging strategy has become common among women. A woman's power may be more tenuous than a man's, and her position is at risk. If another woman chooses to turn on her, she usually can be undercut. It makes political sense to have more than one advocate.

Power Squeezes

The woman manager is in much the same situation. She has fewer power links. She has to carry out the demands of higher-level managers. At the same time, she has to contend with the resistance of employees who resent being stuck in their low-opportunity positions and who are bitter that she got ahead. In order to sabotage her, they may engage in passive-aggressive actions, such as slacking off and not being available. Her response to these actions may make her look demanding, critical, and pushy. These reactions help to perpetuate the cycle as additional hostility and resentment lead to more criticism and efforts to dominate.[19]

The basis of this problem is that women have much less power than men. Until there are several generations of women in power, and until a norm is established, women will have more difficulty handling their power. An environment is created that encourages women to undermine other women. The same dynamics contribute to the unethical actions of men, but women have a much smaller arena in which to play. Women's targets are usually other women, because women are less powerful and less likely to fight back.[20]

Different Management Styles

Women in management positions tend to use a more personal management style. Coupled with the discrimination and opposition that they may have experienced in the workplace, it can enhance and contribute to sabotaging behavior.

The good news is that women managers are more likely to be concerned with the feelings of others. The bad news is that women often lack the political savvy that men have obtained through years at the controls. A more personal management style results in a closer interaction with others; people simply feel better about working together on a specific task. But when things get bumpy, closeness can turn into hostility and personal conflict.

Kids at Play

Psychologists say that one of the reasons for differences in management styles may be that men and women, as children, learn to play by different sets of rules. Carol Gilligan has concentrated her work on how children play. She has found that boys tend to play more competitive games with defined rules, while girls tend to enjoy turn-taking games. Through these games, girls learn to develop more empathy with others and regard rules as being more flexible—something they can readily change if the rules don't work. Boys learn to be independent and yet better able to work on a team and handle competition. They can play with their enemies and compete with their friends, according to the rules of the game.[21]

Adults at Work

These learned patterns are carried over into adulthood. If women are more willing to change the rules, it means a more flexible and adaptive working environment when times are good. It can also mean that when things aren't going well, women will not be bound by the traditional rules of the workplace. The result is a manager who may act unethically, changing the rules when it is expedient to do so. If women are less compliant with team play, in the spirit of competition and compromise, they may be inclined toward revenge against a perceived enemy rather than inclined to regard rivalry for a position as part of the work game. Men lean more toward playing by the stated rules, holding back feelings of rivalry for the overall sake of the team.

Another major difference in women's management style is women's tendency to be critical and controlling. It appears to come about because women may feel more threatened when they use their power. Having power is newer to women. They are more likely to face challenges or resentment from those they manage. Their inclination is to control too much, at times not even realizing they are doing so. Another major difference originates in childhood, when little girls are taught to use persuasion and manipulation, rather than direct orders, to get someone to do something. As managers, women tend to retain and use these techniques in dealing with colleagues and employees.

In today's workplace, management leans toward a more personal and participative style, creating a more humanistic and supportive environment for workers. One benefit is productivity and increased loyalty, but this environment can also be a breeding ground for sabotage. Every workplace has difficult people who vent their feelings and hostilities at one another. They are more likely to reinvent the rules, forming them into whatever seems to be expedient and effective at any given time. The combination of a personal, less rule-bound style with the tendency to be tough and even overcontrolling can lead to chaos. In fact, it can be a time bomb that explodes into a no-holds-barred attack when a woman manager feels threatened and goes after the person who threatens her or is perceived as a threat.[22]

Other Voices

Los Angeles Times writer Judith Trotesky has raised this question: "Must Women Executives Be Such Barracudas?" She relates several examples of no-holds-barred attacks. One woman browbeat her verbally, in order to get her to leave a project. Another privately supported a plan but then proceeded to sabotage it for her own ends. After talking to many executive women, Trotesky found they agreed that women were especially tough on other women. Why? "Because," they responded, "if women want to get ahead they have to be very aggressive." Some also suggested that women are trained to be more malicious and plotting, since they are competing for men. As one woman said, "For a woman to get into a position of authority and power, she has to be something of a barracuda."[23]

Unfortunately, this kind of toughness places a woman manager in a pressure-cooker environment. Achieving women must maintain an excellent track record. It becomes a tremendous burden to do whatever is necessary to keep up.

In the 1960s, Garda Bowman, Beatrice Worthy, and Stephen Greyser wrote an article for the *Harvard Business Review*, asking the question "Are Women Executives People?" In their survey of 2,000 executives, split evenly between women and men, both sexes strongly agreed that a woman has to be exceptional—indeed, overqualified—to succeed in management.[24] Almost thirty years have elapsed since this study, and little has changed. Women managers have to be hard and tough to get ahead, but they are criticized if they are too tough or assertive. Observers may view aggressive, successful women as saboteurs, whereas a man who behaved the same way would not be suspect. Some women may use their power in indirect, manipulative ways in order to maintain their positions. For some, it's the only way to survive.

When Men and Women Use the Same Styles

Ongoing pressures and problems occur for women managers because they face a laundry list of stereotypical perceptions and expectations of how they should behave. Carol Ann Beauvais found in 1977 that the members of a work group judged women more harshly when the women acted in a more instrumental and analytical way, a style that is more characteristic of men. They were more positive when women acted in a more expressive way, the expected female style. The reason, according to Beauvais, is that when a woman tries to use a more rational, nonexpressive manner, there is "greater sex role incongruity."[25] Again, little has changed since Beauvais's study.

My continuing research shows that many women feel compelled to downplay their strengths but must display a tough shell in order to shake off the stereotypical view that they are too soft. What they are doing, in effect, is supporting the traditional male business-method view that a rational, analytical style of management is always best—a style that, over time, will most likely be out of style.

Most women say they tend to do best with some form of the participative style of management, and current research supports that premise. Yet women who adopt it, and do what appears to work best, risk being stereotyped, since this is identified as the primary style of feminine leadership. Other observers believe that women do know how to work with people but lack important leadership skills: emotional stability, aggressiveness, self-reliance, analytical ability, and objectivity—all qualities traditionally associated with men. It's no wonder that women managers feel great pressure to perform.

The Balancing Act

Most women who work outside the home are under a great deal of stress. Arlie Hochschild, in *Second Shift*, reports that when women go home from their for-pay jobs, they come home to another shift, but the woman's male partner or spouse usually comes home to a more "rest and recreation" status.[26] Meanwhile, women proceed with the domestic shift—kids, cooking, cleaning, and errands.

Four main areas of stress exist for women, starting with the "second shift." Women are also likely to receive less pay for work equal or comparable to men's, and anger escalates. Discrimination and differential treatment is another reality that builds resentment. Finally, women can be their own worst enemies: as one woman seeks to get ahead, others may attempt to pull her back.

When men begin their career advancement, they commonly find support from their wives or female partners. Domestic chores are tended to. The woman is more willing to be patient with the professional man as he travels on business or puts in extra time at the office. But the woman executive who is married doesn't often have that luxury or support. Much of the time, she still does the majority of domestic work, as Hochschild reports. If single, a woman executive usually discovers that potential mates resent her time commitments. She may have trouble establishing a relationship, or she may decide not to enter into a relationship because she doesn't have the time to develop it.

In a survey published in the *Wall Street Journal,* over 700 female executives, presidents, vice presidents, and CEOs in major companies reported extra home and personal demands. The married women, even those who earned more than their husbands, did more chores at home. The single women typically had to sacrifice outside interests, including personal relationships, to their jobs.[27] This study was done in 1984. Hochschild's study for *Second Shift* conducted at the end of the 1980s showed no difference, and now, in the 1990s, the consensus of the audiences I speak to parallels the conclusions of Hochschild's work. Someday, women will give themselves permission to hire help for domestic obligations. Unless they love housework (and some do), it makes sense to get some help.

What Women Get Is Not What They Are Worth

When it comes to receiving equal pay for equal or comparable work, women are still shortchanged. Women make seventy cents for each dollar a man makes for the same work. Besides the economic strain that this injustice creates, women's self-esteem is impaired. Women work the same number of hours as men do, and they get less pay. This is a key problem for women who are the primary support for themselves and/or their children.

In the study done for *The Confidence Factor,* I found that a group of "accomplished women" felt the amount of money they made had an effect on their confidence.[28] It can be assumed that women who make less may have lower feelings of self-esteem. Those feelings can become a breeding ground for resentment against those who are doing better by making more, including women in management and supervisory positions, or women who are beginning to move up the career ladder and out of the lower-status groups.

Women executives and professionals who feel held back and underpaid also resent others whom they see moving ahead. If they act on their resentment, the victims are likely to be other women: women are more immediately accessible than upper management and other decision makers, and there are almost always more women beneath an executive woman.

Myths Are Not Realities

To counterbalance misperceptions—that women are not serious about their work, or are too "soft"—women feel that they have to appear tough, and this affects the women under them. One woman wrote an anonymous letter to *Vogue* magazine, saying that she had to be rigid and mimic a man in order to survive professionally: "[As] a top executive in an important corporation... I am faced more and more... with the choice between compromising my human values as a woman, and accepting the dominant dog-eat-dog 'bottom line' ethic, the choice between forcing myself to think more and more like a man or being classed as a 'softie' and served up as dog food myself."[29] But that letter is from ten years ago, when attitudes were even more antifemale than they are now. Stereotyping will fade as more women move into and stabilize their positions in leadership—and when women strive to support other women.

Women as Subordinates

Earlier studies, including Marjorie Bayes and Peter Newton's ("Women in Authority"), have found that subordinates often act in various ways to undermine a woman manager's power, and that other women are often the worst offenders.[30] Typical actions designed to challenge a woman's use of power include going over the woman's head to a male authority, purposely disobeying instructions, pretending not to hear directions, and trying to entice a female executive to abandon the authority role. At times, subordinates may challenge the authority of a male manager, but when they do, they usually use the tactic of open confrontation. When they challenge women, their efforts are much more devious. Bayes and Newton describe such tactics as "unacknowledged, subtle and masked"; subordinates use "covert defiance, denial of subordinacy, or various attempts to seduce [a woman boss] out of that role." The perpetrators are usually women who don't like the idea of working for another woman. Through scheming and plotting, they attempt to subvert the woman in the authority role.[31] One reason why there may be so much conflict between women subordinates and their female managers is that women are normally socialized to take the number two position, with a man in the number one position. As a result, many women resist being accountable to other women because they have "been trained to compete with other women for favored positions with powerful men. It seems difficult for women to join in supporting or protecting another woman.[32]

Subordinates may also resist more directive leadership from a woman because they are used to her playing a more expressive and supportive role. They think she should do things that are helpful and understanding, and they feel a sense of emptiness or abandonment when she plays a more forceful role. They may react with anger and resentment.[33]

Both men and women may treat a woman in authority with anger and resentment. Research initiated in 1965 and revisited in 1985 by Charlotte Decker Sutton and Kris K. Moore found that men, more than women, were willing to accept women as colleagues and competent equals. Sutton and Moore later found a slight percentage increase in the number of male and female executives who believed that women are uncomfortable working for other women. On the flip side, the number of executives who believe men would be uncomfortable working for women declined significantly over the twenty years. These researchers feel that adversarial relationships between women superiors and their female subordinates may be developing and expanding for a number of reasons. First, a female boss may be demanding more now of her female subordinates, in order to mold them into competent corporate women. Second, a subordinate not only may resent the additional demands but also may be disappointed that she isn't getting the warmth, support, and encouragement commonly associated with a female boss. Third, female subordinates may suspect that there are a limited number of slots open to women, and so they feel competitive with their female bosses. Finally, there appear to be more difficult conflicts when a younger woman is supervising an older woman.[34]

Sabotage-Savvy?

Women's undermining of other women is not a genetic disorder. It is a learned behavior, created from years of ingrained stereotyping and societal pressures, and it can change. The "Sabotage-Savvy Quiz" (Exhibit 2.1) has two parts and forty questions. Few will be able to answer *no* to every question. Most of us have participated in some form of sabotaging behavior, whether it was taking credit for someone else's work, not speaking up when someone else took credit for another's work, or just passing along everyday gossip. Each of these actions constitutes a form of sabotage in the workplace. You may wish to take the quiz before going on to Chapter Three.

Exhibit 2.1.   Sabotage-Savvy Quiz.

Part I

   To check whether you are Sabotage-Savvy, answer *yes, no,* or *not sure* to the following questions.

	Yes	No	Not Sure
1. Have you ever given a name as a reference, later to find out that the reference gave you a neutral to negative referral?	___	___	___
2. Have you ever felt that information that would make your job easier or clarified has bypassed you or been withheld?	___	___	___
3. Have you ever felt that files or personal items in your office or workspace have been opened or used without your prior knowledge or consent?	___	___	___
4. Has a group of co-workers or friends ever ceased talking or changed a subject when you approached them (assuming that a surprise event in your honor was not being discussed)?	___	___	___

SOURCE: *The Briles Report on Women in Healthcare,* by Judith Briles. © The Briles Group, Inc. 1993. Permission to reproduce and distribute material (with copyright notice visible) is hereby granted. If material is to be used in a compilation to be sold for profit, please contact publisher for permission.

	Yes	No	Not Sure
5. Has anyone ever passed on or exchanged information about you that was untrue?	—	—	—
6. Has anyone ever taken credit for work you have completed?	—	—	—
7. Has anyone ever not acknowledged you or given you credit for work you have participated in or completed?	—	—	—
8. Have you ever been reprimanded or confronted by someone in front of others?	—	—	—
9. Has someone ever threatened you with a consequence if you did not meet and/or support demands that you felt were contrary to your values?	—	—	—
10. Has anyone ever forgotten to give you important messages or phone calls?	—	—	—
11. Has anyone ever made a commitment to do something for or with you and then reneged on the commitment?	—	—	—
12. Has anyone ever expected you to behave, react, or work in a specific way or according to a specific method, without telling you what the way or method was?	—	—	—

	Yes	No	Not Sure
13. Have you ever been with an individual or a group of people who have identified a problem and made the commitment to seek a solution, only to discover that there was no one to support you in "your" problem when you discussed it with the boss?	___	___	___
14. Have you ever been stuck with doing a co-worker's job because she is often late or spends work time doing personal things?	___	___	___
15. Has anyone consistently criticized areas or items of your work without acknowledging or applauding the positive areas?	___	___	___
16. Has anyone ever tried to reduce or destroy your credibility?	___	___	___
17. Have you ever been terminated without cause?	___	___	___
18. Has anyone ever told someone else personal information that you had shared confidentially?	___	___	___

SOURCE: *The Briles Report on Women in Healthcare*, by Judith Briles. © The Briles Group, Inc. 1993. Permission to reproduce and distribute material (with copyright notice visible) is hereby granted. If material is to be used in a compilation to be sold for profit, please contact publisher for permission.

	Yes	No	Not Sure
19. Has anyone ever called or planned a meeting that involved you, your ideas, or your plans, without including you?	___	___	___
20. Has anyone ever lodged a complaint against you to your supervisor or others whom you work with, without first discussing it with you?	___	___	___

If you answered *yes* to any of the above, you have been sabotaged. If you answer *not sure*, the odds are that you have been undermined. If you answered *no* to all of the above, you work in an ideal environment. Congratulations!

Part II

To determine whether you have ever sabotaged another, answer *yes, no,* or *not sure* to the following questions.

	Yes	No	Not Sure
1. Have you ever offered to be a reference for someone and not given a positive reference when asked?	___	___	___
2. Have you ever withheld information, intentionally or unintentionally, that would have clarified someone else's job or task?	___	___	___

SOURCE: *The Briles Report on Women in Healthcare*, by Judith Briles. © The Briles Group, Inc. 1993. Permission to reproduce and distribute material (with copyright notice visible) is hereby granted. If material is to be used in a compilation to be sold for profit, please contact publisher for permission.

	Yes	*No*	*Not Sure*
3. Have you ever used someone's files or personal items without prior permission?	—	—	—
4. Have you ever participated in or led a discussion about someone else and quit listening or talking when that person or the person's friend or colleague entered the room where you were?	—	—	—
5. Have you ever shared personal information about someone that you did not verify as accurate?	—	—	—
6. Have you ever taken credit for work that someone else completed?	—	—	—
7. Have you ever not spoken up when someone else took credit for work that you know he or she did not do?	—	—	—
8. Have you ever confronted or reprimanded someone when others could observe and/or hear your actions?	—	—	—
9. Have you ever intimidated someone with a demand or a perceived threat if she didn't support you when your demand was contrary to her values?	—	—	—

	Yes	No	Not Sure
10. Have you ever delayed passing on important messages or phone calls?	___	___	___
11. Have you ever reneged on a commitment?	___	___	___
12. Have you ever expected someone to behave or react in a specific way to a situation or problem, without telling her beforehand what your expectations were?	___	___	___
13. Have you ever told someone that you supported her, her idea, or her desire to solve a problem and then not spoken up when someone in authority was willing or ready to listen?	___	___	___
14. Have your co-workers ever had to do your share of work because you spent work time on personal matters (such as phone calls, making appointments, or just being away from your desk)?	___	___	___
15. Have you ever directed negative criticism at a co-worker or employee, without acknowledging some of the positive things that she does?	___	___	___

	Yes	No	Not Sure
16. Have you ever put someone down or belittled her authority or presence?	—	—	—
17. Have you ever fired someone without cause?	—	—	—
18. Have you ever passed on confidential information about someone without her permission?	—	—	—
19. Have you ever planned or called a meeting that involved someone else's ideas or plans, and not included her?	—	—	—
20. Have you ever made a complaint about someone without first approaching her with your concerns?	—	—	—

If you answered *yes* to any of the above, you have sabotaged someone. If you answered *not sure*, the odds are that you have undermined someone. If you answered *no* to all of the above, you are a saint. For the record, my definition of sabotage is: the undermining or destruction of personal or professional integrity; malicious subversion; damage to personal or professional credibility. Any of these can lead to the erosion or destruction of self-esteem and confidence.

SOURCE: *The Briles Report on Women in Healthcare,* by Judith Briles. © The Briles Group, Inc. 1993. Permission to reproduce and distribute material (with copyright notice visible) is hereby granted. If material is to be used in a compilation to be sold for profit, please contact publisher for permission.

3

Caution: Women (and Men) at Work

Men do it, women do it, but men and women do it differently. In healthcare, women's sabotaging behavior will definitely be directed toward other women. Mayhem, damage, destruction, betrayal, treachery, and seduction are synonymous with it. Initially, I thought that the increase in sabotage by women reported from the 1987 study to the 1993 study meant that there was increased awareness among women of having been sabotaged or undermined by other women. Awareness is a factor, but so is the economy. With the shakiness of the healthcare industry, fear and concern have increased, and territorialism has become a major factor: "I will do anything to protect my job, and that includes making someone look bad or undermining another." The "other" is likely to be a woman, for the reasons I have been discussing.

In my 1993 survey responses, I found that when women were undermined by other women, those actions included the following:

- Lying
- Spreading rumors about personal matters and professional abilities

- Making comments about a subordinate's evaluation to other staff before conferring with the subordinate who was evaluated
- Stealing research ideas
- Taking credit for another's work, directly or indirectly
- Telling staff not to be helpful to others
- Interviewing people for a job and not telling interviewees that the interviewer's position is the one to be filled
- Advising a friend not to take an "awful" job, and then applying for it oneself
- Before a weekly office meeting, designating someone as "it," the target of gossip and backstabbing before and during the meeting
- Verbally abusing someone in front of colleagues, patients, and patients' families

The Toxic Workplace: Case Studies

Throughout this book, you will hear voices that show the darker side of women—the side that is not nurturing, caring, or supportive. You will read about vengefulness, secretiveness, backstabbing, gossip, behind-the-scenes manipulation, and activities that can undermine a career. You will read about misuse of power, verbal abuse, and other kinds of pain that women inflict and undergo as they try to maintain their sanity in the workplace.

So Eager to Help, So Eager to Please

Sara had the ideal job. She was the director of a successful women's health center, known for its innovative programs for women and families in the community. The center was also an important factor in the financial well-being of the hospital Sara worked for. Ken, her boss, was someone who had come up through the ranks and whose personality was very different from Sara's.

Sara was determined to work hard and make things positive. Whenever she approached Ken, he would listen. When he nominated her for the state's Woman of Achievement Award, an award she later won, she reached a pinnacle of her career. She developed considerable respect for Ken, although there were times she didn't agree with him. She ran things by him, let him know what she intended to do, got his input and feedback, and then implemented the latest program for the center. Ken's policy was to keep an open door.

One week, when Sara was out of town having surgery, Ken's open-door policy became her downfall. As it happened, Sara was a great believer in teamwork. The three primary employees of the women's center were the office manager, the education coordinator, and herself. They all made management decisions and worked closely together. Sara was pleased that she could empower her staff to make decisions that she would stand by. What she didn't realize is that she had empowered her enemy.

One of her teammates, Mary Lou, begged Sara to let her do more. Mary Lou was happy to screen her calls and resolve disputes between other employees. She told the other employees that she was close to Sara, and that she knew she could help them. Initially, Sara thought that Mary Lou was being very helpful. She was very nice and made a great "right hand."

In most communities where there is a women's health center, the director often receives a lot of local attention and press. Sara was no exception to this rule. She was well known and well liked and was viewed as a role model for women in the community.

Sara's power was challenged when she took a few weeks off after surgery and her "right hand" decided she could run the office as well as Sara. When Sara entered the hospital, Mary Lou started a strong campaign to prove to other employees that she could run the office, and that they should align with her. At the same time, Mary Lou told Sara that she was handling various problems and things were running smoothly. She was able to work through problems and solve them, she said; Sara should just get well.

Initially, Sara thought it was others who were creating the hassles and problems that Mary Lou had to solve. Mary Lou was friendly with Martha, another employee. As Sara continued to recover, Mary Lou and Martha began to verbally abuse another employee, who happened to be a neighbor of Sara's. That employee did not want to take advantage of her relationship with Sara, and so she didn't tell Sara about the others' behavior. After three weeks, Sara returned to work.

In her position, Sara was required to attend various meetings and conferences. Upon returning from one, she went to see Ken. Sara found out that he had initiated several interviews with her staff while she was at a conference. Sara confronted him about these interviews, and he responded as follows:

> Well, Sara, I was just trying to nip it in the bud and talk to them. For the most part, your staff really doesn't like you. There are a couple of them, and you know who they are, that are mad at you. I don't know what you've done to make them upset, but they have a folder two inches thick of things that you have done.

When Sara asked about the contents of the folder, Ken responded that they were petty things. The next day, she returned to the office and asked him if he still respected her, trusted her, and still held her in high esteem. After all, this was the same man who had nominated her for an award. He said that he had "all the confidence in the world" in her. He added that she may have made a poor decision somewhere along the route, and that he had made some poor ones himself. Sara said she needed to think about what had been done, and she asked Ken what he wanted her to do. Ken gave Sara a week to work things out with Mary Lou. After that, he said, one of them would have to go, and he would decide who.

After a week, Sara touched base with Ken. She said she felt that her phone was being tapped and her office was bugged. She was being treated with disrespect in front of other employees and patients. She was also receiving letters from Mary Lou, who refused to meet with Sara in Sara's office because she was tired of Sara "harassing" her. Sara wanted to fire Mary Lou, but Ken wouldn't let her.

The following week, Sara told Ken, "You have to do something. I can't work with the woman anymore. You are going to have to make a decision." Three more weeks passed. Sara then gave Ken a memo that said she no longer wanted Mary Lou in her department. Problems continued. Sara wanted Mary Lou removed within three working days.

Then Sara went to a meeting in another state. When she returned to her office on Monday, she was fired.

Many times, when a staff member sets out to undermine and sabotage her boss, her primary motive is to grab the job. Mary Lou didn't get Sara's. A new director was hired instead, and Mary Lou didn't last another month:

> She thought she would get my job. I didn't have a clue why she thought so, as she had no education or training for the position. Within a month, the new director had fired her. Mary Lou had been caught tape recording conversations with her, Ken, and other employees.

Hindsight is always accurate, and Sara says there are two things that she would not repeat: she became too friendly with her employees, and she gave up her power too early.

Mary Lou's initial strategy for usurping Sara's authority and position was covert and indirect. Mary Lou became more overt when she made direct statements to Sara, refusing to meet with her in her office. But she never said directly to Sara or Ken that she wanted Sara's job, or that she could do it as well.

The Disappearing Mentor

Usually, it's not the employee who undermines the employer; rather, it's the other way around. When a manager or supervisor sets out to belittle or undermine an employee, our research has shown, it is primarily from feelings of low self-esteem and insecurity. The boss feels threatened, and the threat can come from a variety of areas: an employee may let others know that her goal is to be the boss, or an insecure boss may be threatened by up-and-coming employees who are talented and may actually be a peril to the boss's position.

Nancy was a regional manager for a large pharmaceuticals company based in Pennsylvania. She began as an administrative assistant to Bob. He was like a mentor, and she learned a lot about the business. Areas of growth where she could expand her career were pointed out to her. He made her his pupil:

> I put Bob on a pedestal. I was his mentee. I was very young and green, and he wanted me to succeed.
>
> Within a year of my starting with the company, one of Bob's direct reports was promoted to another position. He decided that one of his female managers would take the man's place, and Debbie was promoted.
>
> At first she was great. She was strong and competent and had a wonderful sense of humor. I liked and admired her a great deal.
>
> When she was still being considered for the job, she had come into my office and said, "What's the deal here? Am I the token

woman being considered for this job?" She was very forthright. I responded that I didn't know exactly who all the candidates were, but to my knowledge she was the only woman. I also told her that Bob was very impressed with her and that she should take that as a good sign, because he would say that only if he meant it.

After she had the new position, things changed. I was to report to her instead of to Bob. That was fine with me. I saw her becoming my new mentor and was very excited about that possibility.

Later, Bob and I went to dinner, and he approached me about the possibility of my taking Debbie's previous position out in the field, as a regional manager. I told him I wasn't ready and needed to learn a lot more.

At another dinner, this one with Debbie, she took me into her confidence. She asked me a lot of things about working with Bob. She disclosed that she saw some weaknesses and some things that she thought might be somewhat difficult. When she asked if he was a patronizing manager, I said no. I told her that I admired Bob. His shortcomings were that he was a bit of a procrastinator and let things go to the last minute. Debbie encouraged me to take the management position in the field that Bob had offered me. She felt that I was competent and that her district would be in good hands. She would help me. Well, that's all I needed. I jumped in.

Before long, I realized that I was on my own, and that the promised support was nonexistent. I began to feel that Debbie had pitted herself against me. I realized that at any opportunity she would stab me in the back, with any information she could use.

She worked at driving a wedge between Bob and myself. My once close relationship with him, as his mentee was deteriorating. Many times when I sat down with him for performance reviews, the only negative input came from Debbie. I began to wonder who was ranking my performance: my director and manager? Or Debbie, who was second in charge?

The reports and files that Debbie had turned over to Nancy were incomplete. Not having been a manager before, Nancy was unaware of all the requirements and due dates. When Bob asked for a series of reports, Nancy knew nothing about them, much less when they were due:

> Debbie got away with an awful lot. She knew that she had left me in the lurch by not telling me about the things that were required, and which she had not been doing. I could have gone to Bob and ranted and raved, but somehow I didn't think he would hear me. From what I could see, she had snowed him pretty well.

Many times when people are promoted, they fear that their lack of skills will be uncovered. Nancy felt that she was not totally qualified for her new position, but Debbie saw that Nancy was a quick learner and capable of doing the job. In fact, Debbie saw the possibility of Nancy's advancing into Debbie's own position in the future:

> I was literally out there flying by the seat of my pants, learning as I went along and looking to some of my peers for guidance and help in what I should be doing. I didn't get it from Bob, my former mentor, and I certainly didn't get it from Debbie. The only feedback I was getting at this point was that I wasn't doing it, whatever "it" was supposed to be. I felt like I was in a Catch-22 situation but was bound and determined to make it on my own and get through it the best I could.
>
> I told myself that I would treat her and work with her the best way I knew, because she was going to make or break me. It finally dawned on me that I was a threat to her—that she would do nothing to help my career or support it. I learned from my reps in

the field that she had taken them aside in confidence and asked them a lot of questions about me. Fortunately, I had a good reputation and a good relationship with my reps in the district.

I think she would be perfect for the FBI. She has this way about her that makes you want to like her as a person. She wins you over and then starts to probe with questions. Before long, you realize you've been interrogated.

Our research shows that when someone who is in a supervisory position perceives a threat from someone else, either at the same level or below, the most important rule for survival is to align with someone higher up. Debbie secured herself by her relationship with Bob. Nancy felt that Debbie had learned how to manipulate him and take full advantage of his weaknesses. One time, Nancy approached Bob for guidance. She told him that she felt she had a personality conflict with Debbie:

It wasn't getting any better. In fact, it had gotten worse. I told him that if he had any comments that needed to be made about my work, it might be best if they came directly from him. That way, I would hear them firsthand instead of secondhand.

He was very defensive. He trusted Debbie's judgment because she was in contact with me more than he was. He did admit that if her opinion of me was biased or prejudiced, then that wasn't very helpful. Recently, a man who had worked with the company for thirty years retired. He told me that if the company was going to promote individuals like Debbie, he didn't want to be around. He had had numerous run-ins with her.

When a manager feels threatened by an employee, one of the ways to keep her in line is not to give credit for work she has done, or to deny that she did any of the work in the first place. Nancy experienced this with Debbie:

I worked on a task force that had four members—three of us to do the work, and Debbie as the leader. My style is to delegate assignments quickly, and so I just wanted to get in. I began to implement what we were going to do. Debbie wanted to gab and be the center of attention. In fact, she is famous for that. My style was to keep us on track. The three of us ended up dividing the work equally.

As time went on, I would get glowing voice mail messages from Debbie, thanking me for my contributions and saying that my contributions were greater than those of the other two members. She also said that the things I brought to the table were of high quality, very relevant and valid, and that she appreciated the extra effort. She said that she was going to pass all her glowing comments along to Bob.

I did a stupid thing by not saving her messages. When I sat down at review time with Bob, the issue of the task force came up. I expected to hear all these wonderful things about my participation. He informed me that Debbie said that I really hadn't held up my end of the deal, and that I didn't do as much as the other members.

This stunned me. I was told that I had done a great job, and I knew I had. And then Bob told me I hadn't, and I was devastated. I told Bob that I didn't understand: Debbie had given me several compliments and had left them on my voice mail. I was sorry I hadn't saved them, so I could play them back to him.

Finally, though, I thought luck was on my side. The division I was with folded into another division within the company, and I was given a couple of options, including staying on as a regional manager for the new division. I felt that I could finally get off of Debbie's coattails. Unfortunately, she was made the new area director, and I had to report directly to her. Bob was no longer in the picture.

Women are known for hanging on to a job. If you go to your supervisor, or to the supervisor over the person you are having problems with, your options begin to narrow. You can get the word out about your capabilities and qualifications and look for a transfer, or you can get ready to jump ship. Nancy got ready to jump ship:

> I decided I was going to grin and bear it until I could find another job. Then opportunity knocked. The company decided to expand into new geographical regions. Because I had seniority as a manager at the time, I was asked if I would be willing to relocate. I couldn't say yes fast enough. Several regions were offered. I packed my bags, ready to report to a new manager.

The Susie Attack

Insecurities can pop up in any type of setting. When the boss feels insecure and perceives that employees are stepping into her territory, she may act out her frustrations, both indirectly and directly.

Jeannie was assistant director of a research program at a medical school. Susie was the director:

> Susie perceived that I was trying to act as though I was director of the program. At a meeting with an outside agency representative, we talked about program plans and how another group might be able to help, to be a cosponsor of the events that we were doing. After this meeting, Susie told me that she wanted me to come to her office to go over the budget again.
>
> When I got to her office, I had no idea that there was anything wrong, or that she was angry. After working on the budget for about ten minutes, she pulled out a job description. She told me that she was upset about what I said to the other person in the meeting and about the way I had presented myself. Susie accused me of giving the impression that I was heading up the program, when she was the person who was in charge.

I had gone to her office to talk about the budget. I did not know there was a hidden agenda. She really wanted to talk about my job, and about what she did and did not want me to do. She had written a new job description. I felt that she had lied to me about why she wanted me there. She should have just been direct with me, so that I could have had the opportunity to support myself.

My experience had been that we were open with each other and talked about things, especially things like this change in my job description that she was laying out to me. It really angered me. I had been in the community longer and had helped connect her to many professionals she would end up working with and needing for her research and programs. I didn't think the connections I had built up over the years were threatening. I thought they were something we could tap and use for the education department.

One of the things Susie asked me to stop doing was networking. She did not want me to talk to others in the conferences or workshops that we planned. She wanted me to do registration and any detail work, cover for her until she got to the event, and then leave. She would then introduce the program and work with the participants. I had thought that we were going to work as a team, and that she would involve me in areas where I could utilize my skills. When I found out that I was only to be there as a gofer, and that there had never been any intent on her part to include me in developing professional relationships, I felt used.

Like Nancy, Jeannie resolved to grin and bear it and began to look for a new job. She didn't find one until after she had a scary encounter that almost led to a physical fight:

Susie had interfered with something that was my responsibility. I had made a decision about a program's being cancelled and based my decision on the number of people who had signed up.

Normally, we have many women responding to the programs we do. But in this case, we only had ten participants. I had informed Susie that I had to make this decision, and that there was the possibility of cancellation. She took it upon herself to contact the speaker and tell her that there would be no cancellation and that she would be back in touch. She then came to my office. She was furious with me for making the decision to cancel the program.

I explained to her again what I was doing and why the program was being cancelled. She told me to contact the speaker and tell her that the program was still on. I responded that since she had already told the speaker she would be in touch, it made sense for her to make that contact. Basically, she had already taken it out of my hands and had indicated by her actions that she should take care of it.

Her anger was apparent, but I stood my ground. We started getting louder and louder. Finally I said, "I think you need to leave, and we will talk about it later." Susie would not leave, and I finally told her to get out of my office, that I wouldn't talk with her since we were not getting anywhere. She still would not leave, and so I left. She followed me down the hall, right on my heels. I then turned around went back into my office as our secretaries watched the scene unfold.

I closed my door and stood against it so that she could not force it open. But she put her foot on the door frame, forcing the door open and pulling me out. At that point, we were nose to nose. She told me that the deputy director of the program was going to hear about this.

I wish I had called security or had the secretary do it when Susie refused to leave. To this day, that conflict is known as the "Susie Attack." People remember where they were and what they were doing when it occurred. It was obvious to all: she was the aggressor, out of control.

It's been two years since the "Susie Attack." Jeannie reports that it is still extremely painful. Finally, however, she feels she has been able to empower herself after feeling so defeated and manipulated.

Not Letting Go

Sometimes when a boss is put in charge of a totally new area, it's difficult for her to let go of old ties. She is seen as trying to straddle the fence. In the late 1980s, Mary Ellen was hired as program director for a school of nursing. The previous director had been promoted to the office of dean. But the new dean just couldn't let go of the old territory. Mary Ellen describes the situation:

> Everything I did was tied up with her. I wasn't able to manage my program the way I thought it should be done. People had been encouraged to report to her on anything I did that displeased them. It was a horrible thing. After three months, I felt it wouldn't work, and I started to look for other employment.
>
> The same thing seemed to happen at other campuses affiliated with this university. I had a lot of support from the dean at the school of nursing on another campus. She had always been there for me, but at that time she was forced out by a political power play. It was very disillusioning, the way people went behind her back to get her ousted.

As Mary Ellen discovered, sabotage doesn't happen solely at the lower levels. It also happens in top positions. She felt that conflict was not dealt with fairly. The way individuals at higher levels dealt with others was very indirect and behind the scenes.

Promises Not Kept

Insecurity can lead a manager to reprimand subordinates for unimportant or even illusory things: "If I can put you down and make you feel miserable, I'm bound to feel better."

Jill works in oncology. Normal shifts are twelve hours, from 7:00 P.M. to 7:00 A.M. Jill didn't know that her own boss's job was on the line, and that the support she had been offered would eventually evaporate:

> I've been in nursing since 1984. People didn't stay on our floor long, for a number of reasons. Six or seven years ago, we had a head nurse whose job turned out to be on the line. At the time, I was in a master's program, and she chose me to advance along the clinical ladder. After I had completed all the necessary paperwork, she sat on it. It was held for several weeks. I kept asking her what was going on, and she would respond that she was working on it.
>
> It turned out that she was not doing anything. Instead, she was under the gun because she wasn't functioning well as a nurse manager. She had made several poor decisions and never told me that her position was in jeopardy, nor could she pay any attention to my application. So it just sat there.
>
> After she was dismissed, it was given to another person. By then, it was too late. I had missed the due date. The previous nurse manager had never looked at it, nor had she sent it to the committee. I missed out.

When someone has actively sought your participation in a situation, and you have performed the requested task, you feel undermined when she is not there to support you. The sting in this case would have been reduced substantially if communication had been open:

> When a nurse puts in an application to begin the move up the clinical ladder, it augments the nurse manager's position. I think she was doing whatever she needed to do to save her job. She used me and my application as an instrument to help fill her needs. I wish I hadn't got into the situation, because I was very motivated

and I really wanted the promotion. She left me hanging in the wind. She never bothered to come to me and confide that her position was bumpy and that she might not be able to put it through. I was the first person to attempt a climb up the clinical ladder. My success would have enhanced not only my own career but also the reputation of our department.

Welcome to the Floor

Cindy is a practicing RN working in internal medicine. She has been with her hospital for five years, three as an RN and two as a nursing assistant:

Our floor had just received a new boss. The previous one had been fired, and a nurse from the orthopedic floor had been transferred over as the new nurse manager.

I've always prided myself on reaching out and helping new people. When she called me into her office, she said that she knew that women tried to sabotage other women in the unit. I told her I had been aware of that, and she said that she did not want it to be a factor on her floor. I agreed.

At the same time, a new nurse was hired. Previously, she had been a patient in a psychiatric hospital. One of my tasks was to orient her. When I discussed the distribution of the work load, other nurses thought it would be a good idea to give problem patients to the new nurse. I didn't.

The new nurse could not handle the work. She complained, and I was written up. The new nurse was also treated badly by the nurse manager. I had spoken with four other nurses on different occasions, after that had been talked to by the nurse manager. They were crying and had been written up for things they hadn't done. The new nurse eventually quit because she could not fit in, and because of the stress.

It was not long before our new nurse manager's reputation was well known. She had a bad temper and treated everyone like garbage. I remember telling her that turnover on our floor was substantial; people didn't stay around, and we needed more help. All she could do was scream at me and tell me how hard everyone was working to get new help. She accused me of only thinking of myself. Granted, I was thinking of myself, because I did carry a great deal of the work load, but so did the other nurses on the floor. We just didn't have enough help. The hospital ended up closing beds.

Not All Feedback Is Good

Sharon has been in nursing for several years. For the past five years, she has been director of surgical services. After one year, she had her first evaluation. The outcome was a surprise:

I was called into the vice president of nursing's office for an evaluation. It turned out to be the worst one of my career. When I asked for specific examples, she was unable to cite any. I had been given no warning during the year and had never been told that there were any problems. Being given a poor evaluation, un-expectedly, negated any increases in salary for the coming year.

Unfortunately, the failure to support or document a poor evaluation is all too common.

Your Job Is Theirs

When women act out of low self-esteem, insecurity, and fear, the women they direct their actions toward may find themselves in a difficult scenario.

Ursula was a head nurse for her floor but was moved out of her job, without any warning. She got a phone call from the vice president of nursing's office and was asked to meet with her and the new director of nursing. They had some ideas they wanted to discuss with her:

> I went to the office, and the new director of nursing was there. I barely knew her, just her name, as I had not had the opportunity to meet her personally and spend any time with her.
>
> The vice president of nursing said that they had a job they thought I would be good in. She wanted me to apply for it. I responded that I was flattered, but I really liked what I was doing and did not want to move into another position at that time. They replied that maybe they hadn't made themselves clear: they had a position that they wanted me to apply for.
>
> The bottom line was that I had no choice. I was the head nurse and enjoyed my work, but when it finally dawned on me that they did not want me to remain in the unit, I was shocked.
>
> I had been sitting in on interviews with individuals who, I understood, were being considered for director of the unit. All during that time, I was assured that I was doing a good job. At no time did I know that it was *my* position people were being interviewed for!
>
> I was trying to get to the bottom of what was going on, and so I called the vice president of nursing and begged for an interview. She refused to discuss it. The new director of nursing felt that she was really too new to the hospital to take a position on the matter. At the time, being newly divorced with a family to support, I didn't feel I could just say, "Take this job and shove it." I felt that I really needed to get out of there. I began to look for another job.
>
> By the time I found something I was suited for, I had actually developed a relationship with the director of nursing, who took me under her wing and became my mentor. I got a new job, which was structured as a lateral move without any loss in pay.

It was three years before they hired someone else to replace me, going through three other people until they finally found someone to fit in—a man, and not a nurse.

The position I have today is one that I developed from scratch. I have been here nine years. Both the director and the vice president of nursing have left the hospital

Ursula was fortunate: the director of nursing became a mentor, someone who envisioned Ursula's skills and was able to direct them. Too often, however, women feel that a situation is hopeless, that they are stuck and can't escape.

Ursula herself had been accused of sabotaging behavior and was willing to talk about it:

When I was a head nurse, I had a staff nurse who I felt was un-professional in some of her conduct. She would come to work and constantly flirt with the physicians. My main concern was that at times I observed her being disruptive with patients. I felt that she was there more to boost her own self-esteem than to have any positive interactions with the patients and the physicians. I would counsel her, reminding her that she had a specific job to perform.

Rather than put up with pressure from me, she decided to switch to the second shift, staying in the same unit. When the charge nurse on the second shift asked me about her, I told her of my concerns and described some of the behavior I had noted. Unknown to me, this charge nurse and the staff nurse were close friends. The charge nurse repeated my concerns to her friend.

The staff nurse was furious. Letters were written, and a verbal campaign commenced, saying that I talked about personal and private things, sharing information and evaluations with others. I responded that I had and would do it again. I believe that I was not unethical in my behavior, but the charge nurse was unethical in sharing the information that I passed on, manager to manager. In the end, both the charge nurse and the staff nurse resigned.

For Her Eyes Only

Downsizing has become a buzz word. When companies merge, there are changes, often drastic. Employees feel anxious and uncertain. Sometimes difficulties aren't dealt with straightforwardly.

Pearl is an administrative assistant in a Fortune 500 pharmaceuticals company based in New York. She found a memo about herself in a file that was left out in the coffee room:

> Our department had gone through a series of changes. In fact, it seemed like there was some type of reorganization every week. It all started with a merger with another corporation. New supervisors, managers, and other personnel were brought together.
>
> Lydia, one of the secretaries who worked part-time, quit. Lydia told me that she hadn't been able to stand the politics and infighting since the merger. She had found a job with another company, for less pay and less stress. I didn't blame her. It seemed that everyone was complaining, even calling in sick when I knew they really weren't.
>
> After Lydia quit, my supervisor told me that I would have to cover for her post. I was already taking work home—and not declaring any overtime. I have a preschooler and need at least an hour to get to my home in New Jersey. When I told my supervisor that I couldn't cover for Lydia, she wasn't happy. She even implied that if I didn't like it, I could find another job.
>
> One morning, I took a coffee break. No one else was in the office kitchen. By the coffee machine was a bright-red file. It was labeled THINGS TO DO. I assumed that one of the secretaries had laid it down and left it by mistake when she went back to her station.

I opened the file, to identify whom it belonged to. The first page was a memo that identified whom the file belonged to—my supervisor. By her name was the topic of the memo—I couldn't have avoided it. It said, "Memo to Bernie Re: Terminating Pearl." Bernie was the manager of our department. I didn't know what to do and decided to leave the "hot" file on her secretary's desk.

After a few weeks and many sleepless nights, I decided to make an appointment to talk with Bernie. He didn't say much. He gave no support or recognition for the work I had produced and the dedication I had given to the company. And my supervisor was furious with me for looking in her personal file.

After her meeting with Bernie, the stress escalated. Three months later, Pearl declared, "Enough." She now works where Lydia does. Granted, her pay is a little less. But she enjoys what she is doing. She gets off at 3:30 and is able to catch an earlier bus and spend more time with her young daughter. And she no longer takes work home. Pearl figures that she got a raise.

One thing women need to bear in mind is that the job does not love you. Women tend to be loyal to a job, when the job really isn't loyal to them. Women are often in a very unhealthy and toxic environment. It is an environment that, with continued exposure, reduces your self-esteem to nil and can literally make you sick. An unhealthy workplace breeds poor health for its employees, both mentally and physically.

Pearl's supervisor was what I call an Old Bertha. She had been there for a long time and had seniority. It was improbable that she would be moved or terminated in the near future. When these situations develop, upper management often turns away and does not deal with the problem. In the end, businesses lose billions of dollars annually because so many employees decide that employers can "take the job and shove it." They move on to greener pastures, as Pearl and Lydia did.

The Right Credentials and the Wrong Fit

Theresa is a nursing manager in one hospital within a chain of hospitals on the West Coast. She has a B.S. in business and is an RN She is also working on her master's degree in health administration. She was definitely interested in moving up:

> I was up for a promotion that I didn't get. I had all the right knowledge but the wrong degree, at least from the decision makers' perspective.
>
> When I was turned down for the promotion, a competing hospital in a nearby community expressed interest in me. All of a sudden, they stopped calling. I then heard from three separate recruiters for similar positions in neighboring communities, the same position for which I was turned down at my own hospital. I had been told by the recruiters that each of the hospitals wanted me. And then I heard nothing. When the third recruiter contacted me, I said that I had heard from someone else that I was "off limits." The recruiter said that was impossible. But I was beginning to feel that I had been blackballed.
>
> When another directorship opened up at the hospital, I again applied for it. I definitely had the right credentials, but not the right degree. I was turned down with comments from the interview committee, asking when I would get my B.S.N. I told them that I wouldn't. Instead, I was now working on my master's degree. They were startled that I was able to bypass a B.S.N. and go straight to a master's program. It was like if you didn't play by their rules, you weren't going to play in the game. The master's program is wonderful, bringing me a great deal of satisfaction. It

turns out that several of the people who were involved in turning me down for the directorship are now my classmates.

Although Theresa had the "wrong" bachelor's degree when she was being considered for the two promotions, it may well be the right degree in today's healthcare environment. It makes sense for a manager to have a business background. In Theresa's case, as a nurse manager in the operating room, she has a budget in excess of $8 million. Having a little business savvy certainly makes sense.

Bad News

The voices of these women express great pain over these incidents from the past. All the stories turn on a single question: "How and why could someone do this to me?" Most of the women felt that they had done little to provoke the sabotaging behavior. Otherwise, they wouldn't have felt so hurt.

The next chapter continues these voices. From withheld information to rampant displays of verbal abuse, women who work in healthcare suffer from many of the same symptoms recognized in battered women. From a health-oriented perspective, this is bad news.

4

Saboteurs, Bullies, Gossips, and Other Toxic Co-Workers

Downsizing is a catchall phrase for reducing a work force. Some acknowledge it openly. Others sidestep the issue. In reality, any time there is a strategy to change the size of the work force, from expansion to depletion, there is major impact on all players.

All players feel the force. Those who are let go experience fear, anger, and disbelief. Their morale is at rock bottom. Surprisingly, so is that of those who are not cut. They are fearful that they will be let go in the next series of cutback rounds. They can't believe that their environment is as it is, and they are angry—angry that friends have been let go, and that management has little loyalty or respect for years of dedication. At least, that's the perception. Remaining employees can't help wondering when their turn will come. The end result is a loss for all. Management points to reduced expenses, but are they reduced? When morale and loyalty are at rock bottom, productivity slides. Only time will tell the full impact of the downsizing trends of the 1990s.

Meanwhile, everyone is looking out for number one—herself or himself. Confidences are betrayed, discrimination is more prominent, different types of unethical behavior become commonplace, and tongues sharpen.

Many women have reported that verbal abuse is increasing. Some have used the phrase *verbal assault*. Individuals who put down or betray others, discriminate, and act unethically all display bullying tactics. The most effective way to deal with bullies is to be assertive. It's an ideal way to let others know that you stand behind your opinions and statements and that you are not easily plowed under.

More Case Histories

Women who are assertive usually don't get caught up in game playing. They prefer factual information and don't like to waste time. When women assert their positions, both through body language and speech, communications are less muddled.

Through the Camera's Eye

Clear communications are a requirement for building teams within the workplace. Louise should know. She has taught assertiveness training for several years and is a nursing educator for a large hospital.

One of the formats Louise uses in her courses is that of videotaping participants. This is for their own personal use, so they can evaluate how well they apply what they have learned in the course. In order for people to open up and allow themselves to receive a critique from the class leader, it is necessary to offer confidentiality. That was part of Louise's normal practice:

> In my classes, I normally use a role-playing format. The first time I introduced video to record the role plays among participants, I listed a series of behaviors. In turn, I would watch as well as use the camera for different signs that would show assertiveness,

nonassertiveness, eye contact, body position, and tone of voice. They would work up a script with a partner and then role play it. The camera rolled. The purpose would then be for me to sit down with each of them and discuss what I saw, as well as what they saw. Their strengths and weaknesses were pointed out, with suggestions for changes in behavior, so they could be more assertive. Everyone felt the whole process was very beneficial.

Somewhere between the time the class ended and the time I began to make appointments to evaluate the videos with each participant, the manager of the staff came to me and said that each person had OK'd her viewing of the videos. When I asked her if she had talked to the participants directly, she assured me that she had. I then sat down with the manager and showed her the tapes. Now, these videos are very revealing. They show weak areas, especially when you are nervous or hesitant. She made a lot of comments about each of them.

I then began to have my individual appointments. I mentioned to one of the staff that the manager had already looked at it. The staff member was horrified and asked why I hadn't asked her for permission to allow another to see it. I told her that the manager had said that she had already given it. I then went back to each of the people involved with the videos and asked if the manager had indeed sought permission. None of them had been asked, nor would they have allowed her to see them. I then went to my director and said that there was a breach of confidence and told her what the manager had done.

When I confronted the manager, at first she made an offhand comment: "Well, I guess my staff didn't realize I was going to look at them." Then she denied their denial. I then proceeded to apologize to each participant in the class. I told them I hadn't realized that this would happen. Their response was that they were not surprised; that was the way she treated everyone.

I learned a lot from the situation. I felt that I had been manipulated to get information that could be used against individuals within the course. My credibility had been significantly undermined, and I learned that I would never allow anyone to see a video or anyone's work product without first getting direct authorization to release it.

Louise was fortunate that the participants in the course understood the situation. They didn't like it, but the action of the manager came as no surprise.

Confidentiality Is Not Sacred

When inappropriate actions are taken by supervisors or people in higher positions, and when the targets speak up in their own defense, there are usually two basic responses. One is nonresponse: "How dare anyone question my authority?" The other is outright denial.

Barbara is a marketing coordinator for women's services with a hospital in the Pacific Northwest. She has an M.B.A. degree and maintains a high profile within her community. She can recall several occasions when supervisors took credit for work she had done, ideas she had created and put in place. But the one item that sticks in her mind involves what she believes was misuse of personal employee information:

We had just opened our breast center. My supervisor thought it would be a great idea for female employees to have mammograms. I thought she was going to offer it to all employees. Instead, she took it upon herself to identify all women over the age of forty, contact them, and tell them they needed to come in and have a mammogram. This was without even knowing whether or not they routinely had them with other doctors or even hospitals.

It created a considerable disturbance among the employees, who felt that their personal files and their privacy had been invaded. When I brought it to my supervisor's attention that there was a great deal of friction and anger among the female employees, she merely shrugged it off. At that point, I didn't feel there was anything else I could do.

Many of the women respondents to my 1993 survey stated that personal information did not stay confidential. Even when personal information was obtained through a confidential doctor-to-patient relationship, it was exposed to co-workers.

Kathleen is the educational coordinator for a women's care facility in the Southwest. She is an RN working on her M.S.W. degree. Through the years, she has been affiliated professionally with psychologists and psychotherapists. She found that personal information regarding her family background and the way she makes decisions, information she had revealed to a psychologist, had ceased to be private:

I had accepted a position within a hospice environment. My primary goal was to develop a strong cohesive team. One of the team members was a psychologist, Sherri, with whom I had consulted a few years back. Another was a social worker who was close to Sherri.

At first, I welcomed them as team members. As time went by, however, I became uncomfortable and then devastated. I was shocked that Sherri was using information about my psychological makeup, information she had obtained through past counseling sessions. Here I was, the leader of the team, and during meetings they would whisper, talk, and carry on about their own agendas while others were presenting information. They were rude—to me, to everyone.

What mortified me so much is that I had trusted Sherri professionally. For her to use the information that I had revealed during therapy sessions was unethical. Back then, I didn't have the skills or the knowledge that I have today. I was very naïve.

Initially, Kathleen had viewed Sherri as a mother figure; she was "safe"—matronly, nurturing, and caring. Over time, though, there was a shift. Other traits surfaced—Sherri could be stern, authoritarian, dictatorial, even cold. Kathleen said that, like most mothers, Sherri knew all her vulnerabilities.

Now Kathleen was wedged in a power play. Neither Sherri nor her crony, the social worker, had any respect for Kathleen's leadership. They may have had their own agenda, which could have included leading the team themselves. Kathleen believes that neither one felt she had credibility or deserved the leadership position.

Unfortunately, when undermining is blatant, as in Kathleen's case, and is not confronted or understood, it continues unchecked. Today, Kathleen is more experienced and much wiser.

Closing the Circle

When individuals obtain personal information under a professional umbrella and then reveal it inappropriately, they are either unconscious or totally unethical. Unethical use of information is often tied in with envy, power, and low self-esteem.

Jan is the internal communications coordinator for a hospital that has 10,000 employees and over 1,000 beds. She holds two master's degrees, one in nursing and the other in journalism. Jan recalls what happened when she was promoted from clinical nurse specialist to a position in administration. When word went out that Jan had been promoted, one of her peers began to spread rumors:

I was thrilled with my new position. I felt that I had the perfect job. It would use my nursing skills and knowledge, as well as my newly obtained skills in journalism. When one of my peers, a clinical nurse specialist, found out that I had been promoted, the first thing she did was call people and try to find out how much money I was going to make. She called Human Resources, she contacted different administrators, and then she called me.

When she reached me, she used the excuse that other people had been calling her to ask about me. She said people had asked whom I had slept with to get my promotion. Initially I laughed, but then the real clincher hit. I had confided to her that I had breast implants, a fact that I had kept private. She told everybody. My specialty had been plastic-surgery nursing, and I knew a lot of people in that community.

A few months later, a public relations specialist was hired to present a workshop and work individually with Jan for a few days. When he asked her how things were going after her transition from the nursing environment to administration, she told him what had happened. He responded that he wasn't surprised. He said his experience had shown him that when one person moves outside her former circle, the circle closes and excludes her. In a way, this is a variation of discrimination. Moving on, and up, excludes you from prior connections.

The Honored Guest Isn't Honored

Kim made the transition from being an RN to an M.D. She will never forget the going-away party given by her nursing colleagues as she began medical school. It wins the uniqueness award: a party to which everyone was invited except the honored guest:

I was excluded. I wasn't even invited. I knew a party was going on. I was still working in the operating room. They just didn't invite me!

Initially, I couldn't believe what I had heard Kim say. To my knowledge, this was a first. I have spoken to thousands of women over the years, hearing story after story. Some stories were so absurd I couldn't help laughing. Others communicated the teller's deep pain. Kim went on:

> I had worked in the operating room for five years. On my last day of work, I was involved in a very intricate plastic-surgery case. Normally, my shift is over at three o'clock. At that time, I should have gone to the party. That's when it began. At least, that's what I was told later.
>
> No one was sent in to tell me or relieve me, so I stayed and finished the case. It lasted until six o'clock that evening. On my way out of the operating room, I picked up my going-away gift and a piece of cake that was left for me on the desk. I was ready to begin a new life.

Kim, like Jan, had moved from an "inner circle" to another environment. For Kim, as for Jan, one consequence was exclusion and invisibility.

Belonging to the "Wrong" Group

Lynn is a physician specializing in family practice. She felt that she had been discriminated against because she was the wrong color, the wrong race:

> Part of the problem was being an American female and being white. I worked in the Bahamas, which were 90 percent black. My purpose in going there was to work with Planned Parenthood. It had been a pet project of several people there. They had made many attempts to get it started but were unsuccessful.
>
> When I came, it finally got off the ground. Because of my ties with the United States, I was able to get funding. That was okay

on the inside. But, externally, the original committee wanted the public credit. They were openly angry and hostile toward me and others who had been actively involved in bringing funds to the island.

As an observer and participant, I thought the success of the project was secondary to their own personal glory. The majority of the committee was female. They would bicker over small things, from the décor to types of flowers. There appeared to be more cruel and snide remarks from the women than there were from the male members. When men started joining the committee, there was still conflict, but there was not the level of bickering that I had experienced with the women.

It's not that women are incapable of getting things done—to the contrary. But women report that when committees have a predominance of female participants, a lot of time is wasted on the "small stuff." Jobs that eventually get done could have gone a lot faster if people had cut to the chase.

Chairwoman of the Board

Lisa Marie is the marketing director of a women's center on the West Coast. Her primary credential is life experience. Just a few years ago, she was chair of the board of the biggest hospital in her area. Her experience has been that many women don't help each other advance. They are harder on other women, more demanding, and sometimes unpleasant to work with. When they eventually achieve power, many of them feel that they have to behave like one of the guys:

Women try very hard to achieve the place where they think they should be. When they get there, they feel accepted by the male world. In one respect, they do not want males to think they are siding with females, because they interpret that as a weakening in their position. I also see women worry about how something gets done, rather than if it gets done.

My experience has been that men are more apt to give you a deadline. They tell you what they want and leave you alone so you can do it. I think that women are not taught early on that more than one person can be right at the same time, and that things can be accomplished in different ways.

When I first joined the board at the hospital, other women would caution me not to be too aggressive. It wouldn't look good for women. If I had been a man, it would have been assumed that I was acting assertively and decisively. I had a man on the board who would argue with anything that I brought forward, even when I stated it was at the direction of a committee that consisted primarily of men, such as the executive committee. Because the message was delivered by me, a female, he would argue with me, sometimes even insulting me.

As the first woman chair of the board at this hospital, Lisa Marie found herself in a unique position. She did not fit the female stereotype, nor was she male. Yet as she came forward with decisions and recommendations, whether her own or those of a committee, she risked being discounted because she had broken the traditional mold. She was seen as too assertive by some members:

Women sometimes don't accept the fact that you can be soft and caring *and* be assertive. I found that several women envied the position I found myself in, especially at my age, as chair of the board. They felt that they had done all the right things, agreed with the men on the board almost always, and been ladylike, and yet they hadn't been considered for or offered the position. Several of them were older than I.

During my ten years as chair, the hospital made significant inroads into expansion and presence within the community.

Although a lot of the ideas were mine, many of them were brought forward by some of the heavy-duty men, so that it appeared the ideas came from them. That way, the women on the committees would support them.

One of the differences Lisa Marie found between men and women was that, once she had learned the rules, tasks, and whatever else was expected of her, the men accorded her greater respect than the women did. Many of the women still saw her in a competitive mode, as woman versus woman, rather than in terms of her responsibility for the team—the board. Respect was not automatically accorded her when she gained her influential position. It had to be earned:

I found the women to be less supportive. The more I was respected by the men, the more the women became unfriendly and uncooperative. The men, especially the older men on the board, gave me the greatest amount of respect. Once they saw me work, saw that I had learned what I needed to learn and would accept some of their advice and input, I found they accepted me as the chair.

One older doctor on the board was not an ally when I first joined. He openly campaigned to keep me out. When my name was brought up in nominations for vice chairman, when he was the nominating chair, he put everyone's name on the ballot but mine: I was a woman. His son-in-law later joined the board as a trustee. It was with great pride that I heard that his father-in-law had told him sometime later that I was the best chair the hospital ever had.

Eventually, he became my mentor and acknowledged that I had a great deal of value to bring to the board. Once he realized that, he spent hours and hours educating me about the background of hospital policy, about the hospital's responsibility to the community, and about the healthcare industry in general. Ironically, as I became more accepted by the men on the board, the women distanced themselves from me. It was like they couldn't accept the fact that I could do what I did. I believe that my *power* was unacceptable to them.

Don't Get Excited . . .

Cam is a relief nursing supervisor at an intermediate-size hospital in the Northeast. She remembers the time when a new nurse came into her department, a woman she characterized as a "Sherman tank":

> For some reason, I felt that she had singled me out as competition. She likes power and control. I'm not really a competitive person. I drop back. But she wouldn't let up. She continued to needle me, at least when our boss wasn't around. She was very abrupt, condescending at times, treating me like a child. For example, when she was the charge nurse and I stated my concerns about the condition of specific patients, she would minimize my concerns: "Now, honey, don't you think you're getting a little bit too excited?"
>
> Rarely did I feel that I was treated as a professional. I'm not as particular as some of the other nurses on the floor were at that time, so I would clam up and walk away. My primary concern was that I did a good job—that everyone was pink and breathing when I left. Power wasn't my thing.

Whose Credit Is It, Anyway?

When someone takes credit for someone else's work, there is a feeling of betrayal. Sue Anne is a clinical educator specializing in surgery. She has completed her B.S.N. degree and is now working toward her master's. She recalls a time when a colleague took credit for her work, rather backhandedly:

Ten years ago, I was a staff nurse. We were beginning patient education in the hospital. Our surgery nurses would actually go and see pre-op patients after they had checked into the hospital. Because it was something new, I decided that it would be beneficial to develop a training video for the nurses to use.

One of the other nurses, who was in the education department, attended the annual meeting for the operating-room nurses. In the meeting, there was a special section that acknowledged and gave various awards for new educational programs that had been developed. I did not attend this meeting. My colleague took the video that I had written and produced, and she entered it as her work. Not only did she enter it, she won an award!

To make matters worse, another person who attended the meeting was aware of the deception but said nothing. When the plagiarist was finally confronted, she merely shrugged:

No one spoke up. There were no repercussions for this unethical behavior. She is still in nursing, and she kept the award.

Sue Anne's colleague denied that taking credit for Sue Anne's work was intentional. She said that it was such a good video, it deserved to be considered for the award, and since Sue Anne wasn't attending, the colleague might as well enter it. Sue Anne has learned her lesson. She still produces educational videos, but she makes sure she puts at the beginning of each video, as well as the credits, her name as coordinator and producer. Anyone who views her work now knows it is hers.

When Trust Is a Bust

Nicole, an RN, wears multiple hats as an associate professor, director of a university nursing program, and director of a state alliance for nursing. Nicole's hindsight tells her that a former colleague and friend used her:

Anna, a friend and colleague in the nursing field, planned a series of papers with me. One of us was to be the lead author of the first paper, and then we would rotate on the second, and on the third, and so forth. What started with the best of intentions ended in a huge argument. I agreed that Anna could be the lead author the first time around, and then ended up writing more than 80 percent of our paper. Anna, of course, got the main credit. Along the way, it became clear to me that she was more concerned about her own advancement and credentials than about our collaborative agreement.

It got to the point where I didn't feel that she was trustworthy. We were both at different universities and, with this publication, she was able to get the necessary ranking she needed at her institution. In effect, what she received was enhancement of her reputation, which would lead to promotions and more income.

According to the terms of their agreement, Nicole was to receive lead-author credit for the second paper, but it wasn't worth it to her. She refused to continue the collaboration, and Anna lashed out, calling people all over the country and pleading with them to intervene and make Nicole write the next paper:

It was a very bad experience for me. I finally made the decision not to work with her any longer, after she called other professionals I knew, which ended up impairing my credibility. She caused me an enormous amount of embarrassment. Her insensitivity ended up terminating our professional and personal relationship.

Kellie is a nurse manager on the East Coast. She and a peer have similarly structured units that involve budgeting in clinical areas. They function with the same patient population and under the same physicians. Each manages a staff of forty to fifty employees, with departmental budgets of over $1 million. Kellie and her colleague are well respected, and both maintain a high profile within the hospital.

An associate surgeon of long standing was retiring. They both had a good relationship with him and were looking forward to the dinner in his honor:

> We met formally, to discuss how we would present our units in terms of his retirement. We wondered if we should give a gift or make a speech. My counterpart told me that she had met with the chief of surgery, who was organizing the dinner. We were invited and welcome, but in his opinion, it wouldn't be appropriate for us to recognize his achievements; other doctors would be doing that.
>
> My colleague said she told the chief of surgery that it would be fine with the two of us, and that we would get together as department heads and organize something more personal within the hospital, like a luncheon, where we could do our own presentations and gift giving. That seemed reasonable to me, and I agreed.
>
> The night of the dinner, I went down to pick her up. There was a huge gift in her office. When I asked her whom it was for, she told me it was for the retiring surgeon. She said the staff had already collected the money and purchased this gift, and they wanted to give it that evening.
>
> After dinner, she stood up and made a little speech and gave her unit's gift. It quickly became obvious that my unit had nothing. It was horrible. I can't remember a time when I've been so embarrassed in front of 150 people. My entire staff had been invited as well, and they were furious with me for making them look stupid. They thought I had purposely planned this situation.
>
> I stood there with my mouth open, apologizing to everyone and saying that this was not what we had agreed to. I said I had learned just a little while ago that she was going to present a gift on behalf of her unit.
>
> When I talked to the chief of surgery later, I found out that he had told her that it would be fine for both of us to recognize

him and present gifts. I think her motivation was to make herself look good and make me look awful.

Like Nicole, Kellie no longer trusts her colleague.

The Cost of Withholding Information

When Jo, a nurse educator at a large hospital in Illinois, was new on the job, she was asked to do a task that required the printing of brochures and flyers. The person advising (or not advising) her was someone who didn't want her in the position for which she had been hired:

I had worked with this person a few years prior to my promotion. We didn't get along real well, but in this new position, I felt things were going well. I asked her help in planning a flyer, from the layout to where the postage would be placed in the corner, along with the designated bulk-mail description required by the post office. I also wanted her input on other items that would make this a winning and successful flyer, versus one that a recipient would get and throw in the trash. She had a great deal more experience than I had in formatting.

After I put it together and laid it out, I showed it to her. She didn't suggest any changes, and so took it to the print shop. I assumed I would be getting a mockup or proof before the print run started. When the mockup came back, I would be able to fine-tune and then present it for the final run.

I was wrong. The shop called to tell me to pick up the completed run. It was only then, through the input of others, that I discovered that I had laid it out incorrectly, including the placement and description for bulk mailing.

When I confronted the woman about not telling me, her response was denial at first. Then she said she had assumed I knew all about printing flyers.

Not giving colleagues and co-workers information, whether it is requested or not, when the information could enhance their knowledge and skills is definitely a form of sabotage. One of the most common reasons why women withhold information from other women is that they want to appear to know more and be more valuable than others in the workplace.

Compare Theresa's report about some of the women with whom she works, including a nurse manager in the operating room at her hospital:

> There is one woman, who works in orthopedics, whom everyone calls the Ortho Queen. She holds all the information dealing with cases, or with what's coming up, because she is afraid that someone will become better than she is. In my department, we identified five women she has driven out because they refused to work with her. She undermines them, ridicules them in front of surgeons and staff, and refuses to share anything. When she is on duty, things don't run smoothly.
>
> The departments in our hospital are all very territorial. Few talk to each other. We are bringing in experts who work on team building to help us break the gridlock. My predecessor was a "mother superior" type. She ran the place, and no one dared to cross her.
>
> My goal is to do team building and put shared governance in place. The end result is that we should be able to talk to each other. With shared governance, we are now in charge of budgeting and staffing. Nurses select their assignments, and it's very scary for them, because they have never had to do it before. I have been with the hospital for five years, and I'm just beginning to see some changes.

Miscommunication

Melissa is an administrative manager with a large hospital in the Southwest:

I'm a part time nursing supervisor and work a few days a week. If I see something that needs attention, I'll handle it one of two ways. First, I'll talk directly to the person who is in charge, by phone or in person. Second, I'll leave a note, always including my home number, so they can call with questions.

I had observed a staffing shortage that could have caused a great many problems. I wrote a note to the clinical manager, saying that the floor was understaffed and that there was trouble covering it during the night. I encouraged her to request additional help for the afternoon shift.

Two weeks later, she accused me of having a temper tantrum by writing a note singling her out as the cause of the problem; after all, everyone had staffing problems. I responded that I hadn't had a temper tantrum. I was concerned that a floor with twenty-eight patients had only one nurse for the afternoon shift, and it was my job to point this out.

She denied that there was only one nurse, and then she accused me of singling her out. She had asked the staff co-ordinator and the other supervisor if I had written them any notes about the situation. I said that she was the only one I had contacted, because there seemed to be a problem with the way the clinical manager had left the floor, and that she had the ability to deal with the situation. She then went around telling everyone that I had left a note stating that there was a staffing problem, and that she had had to work with the clinical manager to fix it.

The result was that Melissa's reputation suffered. When her evaluation came up, six months later, she was cited for poor communication with her peers. Melissa showed the other woman the schedule, which indeed showed only one nurse for twenty-eight patients, and her manager finally admitted she was wrong. Unfortunately for Melissa, it was too late. The word was already out that she had been wrong, and that she was passing along information that was incorrect.

What You Give Is Not What You Get

Jennifer was a sales representative for a pharmaceuticals company. The company had recently brought in twenty-seven new sales reps, twenty-five of whom were women. Jennifer had been with the company for several years. When asked to assist in a training class, she gladly gave her time. She remembered what it had been like when she started in the field. She would have welcomed input from other women who had been out there and were successful. Jennifer freely gave her expertise, but what she got in return was not what she had expected:

> I spent a week out of my territory, to assist twenty-five female and two male reps in training. When the evaluations came through, I was stunned.
>
> I had worked up several sales scenarios, using different phraseologies appropriate for doctors, nurses, and receptionists. Role playing was developed, so that they could see how to gain additional information and strategies for closing their sales. When the evaluations came in later, the class assistant told me that this was the class from hell—they gave everybody a hard time.
>
> In the class, there were four women who stayed together all the time, like a clique. They made negative comments on just about everything. On the final evaluations, two women wrote that I was too abrupt, too blunt, and too aggressive. They also threw in that I had wasted their time, and they felt that I was there to pursue my own goals instead of theirs.
>
> I didn't really have to participate in the training, but there was a lot of pressure from colleagues of mine, who felt I could help these women achieve their goals. But their objective seemed to be

to put me down and devalue my assistance. I have heard of similar experiences from other reps, so I feel that my reactions were more typical than not.

Competition

Diane, an admissions coordinator for a hospital in California, felt that she was in competition with a colleague, the director of a medical-surgical nursing department:

> It started a few years ago, when everyone was getting nervous about the direction of healthcare. There were four directors of nursing, and it seemed that two of us were in competition. If I came up with an idea or made a decision, my colleague would counter it, sometimes even telling me never to do something again. After meetings, I found out later, the other three directors would discuss the way I had acted or discuss how my facial expressions were, or even my state of mind: "She seemed to be far away," or "She wasn't responding."

Some of these things may seem minuscule, but when someone is being undermined, the work is often done in bits and pieces—a gradual nudging over, until suddenly the victim is off course.

Leaving Is Not Rejection

When a woman makes a decision to leave a position, the people she leaves behind may feel betrayed. Roz, now a sales representative with a pharmaceuticals company, had been a manager in women's healthcare. When she turned in her resignation, her boss made her last few weeks miserable:

> All the time I had worked there, she had been very compli-
> mentary. We had done several great things together, and I had
> expanded the position I held. I was quite optimistic about the

women's health program, and I knew that with her guidance and management it would continue to grow.

When I turned in my resignation, I gave her two weeks' notice. I thought she would be pleased that I was achieving one of my goals. Instead, she began to throw obstacles in my way that prevented an easy transition out. I feel that she felt threatened. As I got closer to my final days, she kept backing away from me. I think she felt that I had betrayed her.

I told her that I wasn't leaving because I wasn't happy. I had always wanted to work in the pharmaceuticals area, and the opportunity had finally opened for me. She would not talk to me the rest of the time I was there. I had several weeks of vacation coming, and she attempted to reduce the amount allocated. I then had to go to Human Resources to reinstate it. Normally, an exit interview is done, but not in my case. She also refused to give me a copy of my final evaluation.

She refused to see me when I tried to make an appointment to sit down with her. The purpose was to go over some aspects of my job, so that she would have all the necessary information when she decided to fill the position. Instead, she insisted that everything be put in writing.

Women Take Money, Too

Money is definitely a factor in sabotaging behavior; 11 percent of the respondents to our 1993 survey stated that they had lost funds when they were undermined. Ellen has been practicing internal medicine since 1979 in the Midwest. She had an office manager who "borrowed" money:

My office manager worked poorly, hid things, and borrowed money without asking or telling me. When it was discovered that

$10,000 was missing, I confronted her and then fired her. I ended up writing it off on my corporate tax return, and she declared bankruptcy.

Women who were not doctors also stated that they had lost money through loss of a job—being fired, or missing a promotion. It was the women doctors who were subject to embezzlement, as Ellen was. Ellen also is quick to add that she has had good experiences with other women in her office. She had two secretaries for over ten years (both left when they married), and she has nurses who have been with her for several years. One, who had been with her since the opening of her office, died recently.

Margaret has practiced internal medicine for thirteen years in Houston. She too had a problem with an office manager who wrote checks, paid bills, and falsified accounts. Margaret discovered the employee's theft early on:

The woman I hired was the ex-wife of a doctor. She was using drugs. After I discovered the embezzlement, I spoke to her ex-husband. He told me that he also thought she had embezzled from him, but it's very difficult to prove when the embezzler is your wife, and he certainly couldn't take her to court.

I knew something was wrong after the first month she was here. She paid the bills and used my stamp to falsify checks and accounts. At the time she was fired, $18,000 had been taken. I elected to prosecute, and the court put her on probation and ordered her to reimburse me at the rate of $45 per month.

Note that both Ellen and Margaret confronted their employees. It will take Margaret a long, long time to recover her funds, but she is committed to following through and letting others know, so they can avoid the same situation.

Women in Charge

Control, or lack of it, is an important issue for a lot of people. Peggy, a partner in a family practice in Connecticut, was a medical student when she encountered a woman who needed to be in control. This woman specialized in giving female medical students a hard time:

> I was in my fourth year of medical school, in a rotation known as a subinternship. It is similar to an internship, but with a great deal of supervision.
>
> It was normal to get one admission a night, which we would write up with a series of orders, and the resident would then cosign it. The official rule is that the subinterns are not supposed to write orders, but the unwritten rule is that if the orders are reasonable, the nurses look the other way and even follow them before the resident has the opportunity to sign.
>
> There was one nurse who was like Nurse Ratched in *One Flew Over the Cuckoo's Nest*. She was miserable to the women students. I had a patient in acute congestive heart failure, and I needed to get some medicine to him. She would not honor my orders or listen to me. I had my orders cosigned, but the nurse snatched them up without looking at them. Then she demanded that I get them cosigned. When I brought it to her attention that they had already been cosigned, she just stomped off in a huff.

Robyn has a family practice in New Mexico. She recalls a nurse who didn't like her:

> When I first got out of my residency, I worked in the emergency room in Santa Fe. There was another female physician who had a good reputation and was well liked. With a woman doctor already ahead of me, I felt that my transition would be much easier.
>
> I was wrong. The head nurse decided she didn't like me. She

told the other nurses not to help me. When I had a patient who needed stitches or something cleaned out, the nurses would disappear. I would end up doing everything myself. I wouldn't have known I was the head nurse's victim if one of the nurses who liked me hadn't pulled me aside and told me that the head nurse had instructed them not to help me.

The head nurse had been around for more than twenty-five years. Eventually, I concentrated on growing a family practice, and I moved on.

"Horizontal Violence"

Laura Gasparis Vonfrolio is presently working on her doctorate and has certifications in critical care and emergency room nursing as well as a master's degree. She is the publisher of a quarterly journal called REVOLUTION— The Journal of Nurse Empowerment, a nursing journal that's not quite like any mainstream nursing journal. Articles from REVOLUTION include "Should Nurses be Counseling on Condom Use?" "Can This Marriage Be Saved (Contemplating a Divorce from Nursing)," "Media Watch: Television Coverage of Health Care/Can Nurses Break In?" It's not uncommon to find prewritten, tear-out postcards addressed to the president of the United States, 60 Minutes, or Oprah Winfrey in an issue. The purpose is to make communication to decision makers and personalities about nursing as simple as tearing out the card and putting a stamp on it.

Gasparis Vonfrolio believes that hospitals pit nurse against nurse by establishing such systems as primary nursing, "shared governance," and "career ladders."

According to her, primary nursing eliminates nurse aides and licensed practical nurses (LPN). Highly trained RNs, regardless of professional level, now deliver lunches and empty bedpans and trash.

Many hospitals rationalize the elimination of aides and LPNs as a cost reduction measure.

Shared governance and career ladders surfaced in the last decade. Initially, many felt that when shared governance became popular and nurses were put in charge of their own budgeting and staffing, it would have a positive effect. Unfortunately, with budgets continuing to shrink, nurses end up grumbling among themselves about over-time and work loads. Career ladders are associated with teamwork. Many nurses feel that when one team gets a reward, it's usually at the expense of another.

Gasparis Vonfrolio feels that the demeaning of nurses begins in nursing school (where most nursing professors do not practice nursing). She says:

> Several years ago I did a study comparing the perception of students in nursing and students in medicine. I visited the first day of school in several parts of the country. The common phrase that came from all the schools of nursing to beginning students went something like this... "Look around you; only half of you are going to make it."
>
> This was quite a departure from what I heard from the medical schools. In medical school, as each student passed through the door to the first orientation meeting, the professor stood at the door shaking hands, greeting them and addressing them as doctor. They were no more doctors than my mother was. My thought was, "So this is how it all starts."
>
> The first day of nursing school, the women are told that only half are going to make it, but in the predominately male medical school the professor is standing at the door assuming that all will make it.

When individuals in a group feel oppressed and suffer a lack of or de-cline in self-esteem, they are more likely to undermine one another.

Gasparis Vonfrolio believes that nurses are an oppressed group. Although they flock together, they don't stick together. When she talks about hospitals pitting nurses against each other, she uses the phrase "horizontal violence." Because of this horizontal violence there are times when a patient's life may be in jeopardy. In a situation where a patient is hemorrhaging, the floor is short staffed, a nurse needs help, and the only person who is available isn't among her friends, the odds that the other nurse will help in a timely manner are greatly reduced.

Verbal Abuse...Alive and Deadly

In the early eighties, S. B. Freidman did a study focusing on re-lationships between nurses and physicians. She concluded that nurses were subjected to condescension, temper tantrums, scapegoating, and public humiliation at the rate of six occurrences per month per nurse. In 1987, Helen Cox, the Associate Dean of Continuing Nursing Education at Texas Tech University Health Science Center for the School of Nursing in Lubbock, Texas, released her findings on verbal abuse among nursing personnel. The purpose of her study was to identify the frequencies, sources, nature of impact, and possible so-lutions for verbal abuse. According to the study, these kinds of con-flicts between nurses and their peers and between nurses and both top level administrators and nursing administrators contributed more to nurses burning out and leaving the profession that any other factors. She found that 82 percent of staff nurses reported experiencing verbal abuse. The perpetrators of the abuse in order of "rank" were: physicians, patients, families of patients, and immediate supervisors.

Verbal abuse, whatever the cause, has a negative effect on every-one. Verbal abuse of nurses has been linked to feelings of powerless-ness, incompetence, and low self-esteem and self-worth.

In a follow-up to Cox's work, Kathryn Braun, Donna Cristle,

Dwayne Walker and Gail Tiwanak of the Queens Medical Center in Honolulu, Hawaii, decided to survey all registered nurses employed by the hospital in mid-1989 using Cox's original survey questionnaire. Nurses again reported six or more abusive situations a month, with 80 percent of the staff reporting abuse from patients, 78 percent from a physician, 60 percent from a patient's family, 52 percent from staff nurses, 24 percent from immediate supervisors, 21 percent from subordinates, and 6 percent from administration.

Suzanne Zigrossi, who heads the Women's and Children's Center at Baptist Hospital in Miami, Florida, found in a study that the predominant abuser was the patient, followed by the patient's family, physicians, peers and then supervisors—a slight variation from what Cox found. Types of behaviors included anger, disapproval, belittling comments, obscene language (usually from patients), name calling, rudeness, unreasonable demands, physical threats, sarcasm, sexual suggestions, condescending behavior, and ridicule.

Are Nurses Battered Women?

A common reaction to abusive behavior is reduced self-esteem and self-worth. If nurses, 97 percent of whom are women, report they experience verbal abuse six times a month, it is not surprising if low self-esteem results. Many of the women interviewed for this book compared the experience to that of a battered woman.

In 1979, Lenore Walker published her ground breaking book *The Battered Woman*. In it, she said the typical battered woman has a poor self-image and low self-esteem. Battered women base their feelings of self-worth on their perceived capacity to be good wives and homemakers. If they have successful careers outside the home, they are secondary. If you take Walker's description of a battered woman and change just a few words, it fits the feelings of many women in the nursing profession.

The typical *abused nurse* (battered woman) has a poor self-image and low self-esteem, basing her feelings of self worth on her perceived capacity to be a good *nurse* (wife and homemaker), whether or not she has successful *career* (life) within her *workplace* (home).

Words Are Harmful

Many nurses said that one sabotage particularly painful to them is gossip, especially malicious gossip. Mary Ellen, who has been in the field of mental health for many years, said she knew that everyone around the world gossips, but in nursing it is particularly bad.

Naomi, director of a women's health floor in a hospital with 500 beds, looks back at the time when she was clinical nurse specialist in obstetrics. She remembers the gossip factor all too well. She feels that there is no worse gossip than what is heard on an OB floor:

> A lot of gossip was around sexuality and sex. Some of the jokes were funny. I wasn't married, nor was I dating at the time. I'm straight and had never done anything to indicate otherwise, but I was the butt of jokes on my floor. I remember one time a nurse came up to me and said, "Naomi, you're just like the slogan for 7-Up: you never had it, and you never will." And then she started laughing out loud in front of ten other women in our department. I was so angry and stunned, all I could do was cry.

When people aren't busy, they have more time for whatever it is they want to talk about. Naomi suggested that this could be a factor with OB nurses: there are times when they are intensely busy, and times when babies aren't being born. Idle time is perfect for gossip.

Sue Anne agrees with Naomi. She works as a clinical educator in surgery and is aware of the closeness of the operating-room personnel. When we asked if she had any preference in terms of working with men or women, she had none. But then she added that women "gossip and tear each other apart." It infuriates her:

> I work in several different operating rooms. Each is a close-knit group of women, most of whom, I found, don't want to confront a situation, especially if it's ugly. When someone is angry, the prevailing style is not to go directly to that person and try to resolve it. Rather, it's to talk to someone else, which eventually has the whole unit buzzing about whatever it is that happened. It's heard at second, third, fourth, fifth, and tenth hand and blown all out of proportion. If I have done something, I want to hear about it now, not six months down the road.

The "It" Girl

Kimberly is now an administrative secretary at a women's resource center in a hospital located in the South. Here is what she says about the time when she worked for another hospital:

> I did primarily clerical work at the hospital. It was small quarters, and each week we would have a meeting. I hadn't been there too long, but it seemed to me that each time we got together, a person would be picked on. Initially, I didn't pay much attention. They were nice to me, but after a while I became the current "it."
>
> The manager, and a couple of other people who were her close friends, selected someone early in the week. Throughout the week, they treated her coldly and with indifference, even making the job a little harder on her. They would start to let personal comments slip out, which would eventually lead up to the meeting on Friday—the grand finale.
>
> By the time we got to the meeting, the managers would say something like "We need to discuss the problems we are having

with Joanne" or "Let's identify some problems that Joanne is having." Then everyone would be free to make comments. I'll never forget the time it was my turn to be "it." Someone made comments about my hair and how I really needed a perm. Then another woman in the group acknowledged the first commentator, saying that I did need to do something about my hair. Someone even offered to pay for the perm!

I remember one time when another woman was "it." She had been there longer than I had, and the group started to talk and say things about her being slow and not moving fast enough, and about her starting to gain weight. She'd had it, and she was ready for them. She pulled out her resignation, already typed, and dropped it on the table. Then she walked out.

Kimberly also left that workplace eventually. Leaving is always an option—usually not the first choice, but one that should be considered early in a deteriorating situation. The prospect of leaving should not be used as a threat to the saboteurs, at least not initially. Rather, it should serve as a personal option, to be put into play if the situation doesn't change.

Contagious Negativity

Deteriorating situations exude negativity, and negativity is always on the lookout for a new home. It is easy to absorb someone else's negative energy. And once negativity has infected a deteriorating situation, its impact seeps into every corner of the workplace, adding to the toxicity.

5

The Art of Constructive Confrontation

Conflict and confrontation should go hand in hand, and many women realize that they ought to confront a saboteur directly. After all, when there is no confrontation, sabotage goes unchecked. So why do women so rarely engage in direct confrontation? The answer is found in an old dictum: "Nice girls don't complain."

Anger and Conflict: Misconceptions

Many people believe that the sign of a poor manager is the development of conflict. Some believe that a conflict signals low concern or support on the part of management. Many believe that anger is destructive, while others believe that if you leave a conflict alone, it will go away. There is also the belief that all conflicts must be resolved, no matter what; smile, shake hands, and let bygones be bygones.

All these beliefs are misguided. Conflict arises in the workplace because people have different goals and objectives. Their perceptions vary. They hear differently. Culture, race, and gender all play a part. There is also general "noise"—news, events, fear, and concern—that creates conflict. Most conflicts are believed to be rooted in some specific action or context. In reality, however, they are usually caused by communication failures or breakdowns, specifically in listening.

There are times, of course, when conflict results from deliberate provocation. When you can identify a situation in which another is purposely trying to hurt you, my advice is to get out. You are not going to change this person, and you will not have time to go through the series of processes that might enlighten her. Most of the time, though, a saboteur is out to enhance her own reputation, and you just happened to be in the way.

Because women are inclined to have "confrontophobia," what seems to be a primary conflict may actually be an accumulation of half-remembered and relatively minor items, which can magnify a problem the size of a gnat into a problem the size of an elephant.

Characteristics of Conflict

As a conflict escalates, concern for oneself increases. The desire to win increases in turn with the rise in self-interest. Saving face takes on more importance as a conflict builds.

Conflict-management strategies vary: what works at a low level of conflict may be ineffective or counterproductive at a higher level, and people may use different styles of conflict within a conflict. When you are dealing with someone you must confront, personally or professionally, it makes sense to identify her strengths and weaknesses by understanding her preferred style of handling conflict. This means you have to step back, put yourself in her place, and try to anticipate her responses and reactions.

Styles of Managing Conflict

Sometimes a particular conflict-management style will work best in a specific situation. Ideally, you should be able to recognize which conflict styles are emerging when you are dealing with someone, as well as the style or styles with which you are responding. As you become more skilled in dealing with conflicts, you will be able to choose the conflict-management style that is most appropriate.

One of the first steps is to discover what your preferred style of managing conflict is, and Exhibit 5.1 will help you do that. Figure 5.1 displays five modes of managing conflict—competing, collaborating, accommodating, avoiding, and compromising—along two axes, one that represents assertiveness and one that represents willingness to cooperate. Below, circle the response that best reflects you.

Exhibit 5.1. Conflict-Management Style Survey.

1. When you have strong feeling in a conflict situation, you:
   A. Enjoy the emotional release and sense of exhilaration and accomplishment.
   B. Enjoy the challenge of the conflict.
   C. Become serious and concerned about how others are feeling and thinking.
   D. Find it frightening because someone will get hurt.
   E. Become convinced there is nothing you can do to resolve the issue.

2. What's the best result you can expect from a conflict?
   A. Conflict helps people face facts.
   B. Conflict cancels out extremes in thinking so a strong middle ground can be reached.
   C. Conflict clears the air and enhances commitment and results.

SOURCE: National Businesswomen's Leadership Association, a division of Rockhurst College Continuing Education Center, Inc. Reprinted by permission.

    D.   Conflict demonstrates the absurdity of self-centeredness and draws people closer together.

    E.   Conflict lessens complacency and assigns blame where it belongs.

3. When you have authority in a conflict situation, you:
    A.   Put it straight and let others know your view.
    B.   Try to negotiate the best settlement.
    C.   Ask for other viewpoints and suggest that a position be found that both sides can try.
    D.   Go along with the others, providing support where you can.
    E.   Keep the encounter impersonal, citing rules if they apply.

4. When someone takes an unreasonable position, you:
    A.   Lay it on the line and say that you don't like it.
    B.   Let him or her know in casual, subtle ways that you're not pleased, possibly distract with humor, and avoid direct confrontation.
    C.   Call attention to the conflict and explore mutually acceptable solutions.
    D.   Keep your misgivings to yourself.
    E.   Let your actions speak for you, possibly using depression or lack of interest.

5. When you become angry with a peer, you:
    A.   Explode without giving it much thought.
    B.   Smooth things over with a good story.
    C.   Express your anger and invite a response.
    D.   Compensate for your anger by acting in opposition to your feelings.
    E.   Remove yourself from the situation.

6. When you find yourself disagreeing with other members about a project, you:

    A.   Stand by your convictions and defend your position.

    B.   Appeal to the logic of the group in the hope of convincing at least a majority that you are right.

    C.   Explore points of agreement and disagreement, then search for alternatives that take everyone's views into account.

    D.   Go along with the group.

    E.   Do not participate in the discussion and don't feel bound by any decision reached.

7. When one group member takes a position in opposition to the rest of the group, you:

    A.   Point out publicly that the dissenting member is blocking the group and suggest that the group move on without him or her, if necessary.

    B.   Make sure the dissenting member has a chance to communicate his or her objections so that a compromise can be reached.

    C.   Try to uncover why the dissenting member views the issue differently, so that the group's members can reevaluate their own positions.

    D.   Encourage members to set the conflict aside and go on to more agreeable items on the agenda.

    E.   Remain silent because it is best to avoid becoming involved.

8. When you see conflict emerging in your team, you:

    A.   Push for a quick decision to ensure that the task is completed.

    B.   Avoid outright confrontation by moving the discussion toward a middle ground.

C. Share with the group your impression of what is going on, so that the nature of the impending conflict can be discussed.
D. Relieve the tension with humor.
E. Stay out of the conflict as long as it is of no concern to you.

9. In handling conflict between group members, you:
A. Anticipate areas of resistance and prepare responses to objections prior to open conflict.
B. Encourage your members to be prepared by identifying in advance the areas of possible conflict.
C. Recognize that conflict is healthy and press for the identification of shared concerns and/or goals.
D. Promote harmony on the grounds that the only real result of conflict is the destruction of friendly relations.
E. Submit the issue to an impartial arbitrator.

10. In your view, what might the reason for the failure of one group to work with another?
A. Lack of a clearly stated position or failure to back up the group's position
B. Tendency of a group to force leaders to abide by the group's decision, as opposed to promoting flexibility, which would facilitate compromise
C. Tendency of groups to enter negotiations with a win-lose perspective
D. Lack of motivation on the part of one group's members to live peacefully with another group
E. Irresponsible behavior on the part of a group's leaders, resulting in the leaders' placing emphasis on maintaining their own power positions rather than addressing the issues involved

Now total the number of A's, B's, and so on, and insert below:

A _____ B _____ C _____ D _____ E _____
Competitive   Compromise   Collaborative   Accommodative   Avoidant

To score the survey, total the number of A's, B's, C's, D's, and E's from questions 1 through 10. (The scoring system has been modified to simplify interpretation of results.) Remember that it is common to start by using your secondary or backup style of conflict management, then move on to your primary style if you feel you are not being heard or if you are not getting satisfactory results.

Now complete the survey again, this time substituting the pronouns *she* (*he*), and so on, for *you*. You will then have a strong indication of what your opponent's conflict-management style is. This puts you in the driver's seat, allowing you the opportunity to take the lead and adjust your style to match hers. When this happens, she will be better able to hear what you have to say, and a compromise is more likely to be achieved.

Look at the left side of Figure 5.1. You know when you are being unassertive: you want to pull back from conflict, and you will do anything to avoid a confrontation. When you are being assertive, you are more aggressive and active in dealing with conflict. If you speak up for what you believe, or for what you perceive as justified, you are on the assertive side. If you believe that others routinely take advantage of you and that your voice isn't heard, you lean toward being unassertive.

Now look at the bottom of Figure 5.1. If you are a cooperative person, you will do whatever you can to work with another, even when you don't agree with her. If you are uncooperative, either you avoid dealing with her or you attempt to resolve the issue in your own way. When things don't go your way, do you say "I'm out of here"? Or do you say, "Wait a minute. Let's continue working and see if we can get to a resolution"?

Figure 5.1. Five Modes of Managing Conflict.

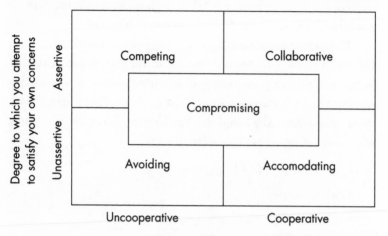

SOURCE: Adapted from the Thomas-Kilmann Conflict Mode Instrument, developed by Kenneth W. Thomas and Ralph H. Kilmann in 1972. ("Mode" is an acronym for "Management of Differences Exercise.")

Competing

When a woman is competitive, her style is a very assertive one. She is primarily interested in getting her own way. She usually is not interested in cooperating with others, and she approaches conflict in a direct and forceful way: "I don't care what other people think, it's my way or none." Women who are predominantly in the competitive mode are most interested in satisfying their own concerns, often at the expense of others, and they will do it by pulling rank, being forceful, and arguing. Queen Elizabeth I, for example, ruled with a very firm hand. She surrounded herself as much as possible with submissive men. She was in charge. It was her game. She made the rules, and others followed. England's queen of today does not have the power of her sister and namesake of yesteryear. The closest female equivalent to Queen Elizabeth I that England has generated in modern times is former Prime Minister Margaret Thatcher.

The competing mode is a good one to have at your disposal when you are in a position of power, but it can alienate people. If you are someone with little power and you use the competing mode in a disagreement with a manager or supervisor, you may get yourself fired. In her book *Resolving Conflict*, Gini Graham Scott lists the times when competing is best. Compete when you:

- Are creating a win-lose situation
- Must use rivalry
- Must use a power play to get what you want
- Must force submission
- Feel the issue is very important to you, and you have a big stake in getting your way
- Have the power to make the decision, and it appears that your way is the best way to act
- Must make a decision quickly, and you have the power to make it
- Feel you have no other options
- Feel you have nothing to lose
- Are in an emergency, where immediate and decisive action is necessary
- Can't get a group to agree, or feel that you are at an impasse and that someone must make the group move ahead
- Have to make an unpopular decision, action is required now, and you have the power to choose what to do

Popularity should not be your primary objective when you are in the competing mode, although you may in fact win supporters and admirers if your solutions work. Competing is for getting your way when something is important to you. When you feel that you have to move quickly or act immediately, and when you are confident that you will succeed, use of the competitive style does not necessarily mean that you are pushy or a bully.

Collaborating

Collaborators are actively involved in working out conflicts. If your style is one of collaboration, you vocally assert what you want but at the same time cooperate with the other person. Being collaborative takes longer because you first have to identify concerns and issues. Then, each party must be willing to listen to the other's needs and concerns, as well as other issues. If you have the time to process issues in this mode, a win-win scenario will probably evolve.

Collaborating may initially seem appropriate when parties say that their goals are the same. There may be underlying disputes, however, and sometimes there is confusion about what the overall goal is.

For example, a woman is consistently late to work and spends a lot of work time on personal business. Getting her to cut back on her use of the phone or keep track of how many minutes she spends on personal business doesn't solve the problem, and she begins to act out in other ways. You want her at work on time, and you want her to do her work, not take care of her personal business. That's your goal, and it may actually be hers, too. But something is blocking her commitment. Is she bored? Does she feel unappreciated? By actively listening, and by eliminating or dealing with obstacles presented by her, you will move closer to your goal. In fact, the mode of collaborating often encourages each party to identify her needs and wishes. Collaborating works best when you:

- Are in a problem-solving position
- Confront differences in sharing ideas and information
- Search for integrated solutions
- Find situations whereby both of you can win
- See problems and conflicts as challenging
- Know that the issues are very important to both parties
- Have a close, continuing, or interdependent relationship with the other party
- Have time to deal with the problem
- Know you and the other person are aware of the problem and are clear about what you both want
- Are confident that the other party is willing to put some thought and work into finding a solution with you
- Both have the skills to articulate your concerns and listen to what the other has to say
- Both have similar amount of power or are willing to put aside any power differences in order to solve the problem together

Collaborating takes time, work, and a lot of effort. It can be an excellent, amicable approach to getting needs and issues recognized and met. Everyone involved must commit time, be able to clarify wishes and needs, be willing to listen to others, and be willing to explore alternatives and agree to a solution. Otherwise, collaborating won't work. But when it does work, it can be the most satisfying resolution for everyone, especially in a serious conflict.

Accommodating

The person in the accommodating mode likes to help. Often she is someone who conforms easily. Accommodating means cooperating without asserting one's own claims to power. It works well when the goal is not very important to you. When you have decided that you are in a no-win situation, it makes sense to be accommodating; you might as well go along with whatever the other person wants. The accommodating mode is also appropriate when your strategy is to smooth things over for now but bring the issue up again later. This is deferral, not avoidance. If you feel that accommodating would mean giving up something important, then the accommodating mode is not appropriate.

Accommodate another when you:

- Want to give way
- Wish to submit and comply
- Don't really care what happens
- Want to keep the peace
- Feel that maintaining the relationship is most important
- Recognize that the outcome is more important to the other person than to you
- Recognize that you are wrong
- Have minimal or no power
- Have no chance of winning
- Think the other person may learn from the situation if you go along with what she wants, even though you do not agree with what she is doing or think she is making a mistake
- Want to learn more
- Want to show that you are a team player

- Want to collect favors, to be redeemed later
- Want to minimize certain loss

When an environment is negative or hostile, harmony can often be restored by accommodation. By sacrificing your concerns and yielding to what another person wants, you may be able to smooth over a bad situation and use the period of calm to gain time. In the end, you may be able to work out a resolution that you would like more.

Avoiding

The avoiding mode is similar to accommodating. You use it when you feel that you are in a no-win situation, when you don't want to be a bother, or when the whole problem or issue is of little or no importance to you. You also use it when the other person has more power or may be right, or when it is not worth your time to take a position. This mode is one of sidestepping and ignoring the issue or delaying input or decisions. It can work temporarily when you are dealing with someone who is difficult and there is no need for you to work together. You make the choice to not make a decision.

The problem is that if you don't come back later to deal with the issue, others may view you as a procrastinator or as irresponsible. If deferral is your real objective, eventually you have to come back and deal with the issue. Use the avoiding mode when you:

- Want to ignore a conflict, or hope it will go away
- Want put problems on hold
- Want to slow things down and stifle a conflict
- Want to use secrecy to avoid a confrontation
- Want to appeal to bureaucratic rules
- Sense that tensions are too high, and you feel the need to cool down or back off

- Believe that the issue is trivial
- Are having a bad day, and there is high probability that you will get upset and not deal logically or rationally with the situation
- Cannot win and know it
- Want or need more time, either to gather information or to get help
- Know that the situation is complex and difficult to change
- Feel that any time spent on the problem will be a waste
- Have little power to resolve the situation or find a beneficial solution
- Feel that you aren't qualified to resolve the situation, and that others can do better
- Know that the timing is bad, and that bringing the conflict into the open may make things worse
- Want to let people cool down and regain perspective

Avoiding doesn't necessarily mean being evasive or running away from an issue. There are times when evasion or delay is appropriate and constructive, and some conflicts really do resolve themselves if they are left alone.

Compromising

In the compromising mode, you give up some of what you want to get the rest of what you want, and other parties do the same. The solution, by definition, doesn't satisfy any one party completely, but it does meet the majority of each party's concerns and objectives.

One of the differences between collaborating and compromising is that in collaboration you search for underlying needs and interests;

in a compromise, each person gives up some of those needs and interests before a resolution is reached.

Let's say you and a co-worker both want the Christmas holidays off. You each have the same objective, yet only one of you can have what you want. As a compromise, one of you can work on Christmas Eve, and the other can work on Christmas Day; or one gets Christmas off this year, and the other gets Easter. Whatever the solution, neither of you is going to be 100 percent satisfied, because neither of you will get everything you want.

In a compromise, conflict is a given. What you seek is a way to change the conflict into an exchange. In collaboration, a long-term win-win solution is often the goal; in a compromise, the outcome is more likely to be short-term and expedient. At the end of a compromise, the normal response from both parties is "I can live with it." Use compromise when you:

- Need to negotiate
- Are looking for deals and trade-offs
- Want a satisfactory or acceptable solution
- Have power equal to your opponent's, and you are both committed to mutually exclusive goals
- Want to achieve resolution quickly
- Need to save money
- Are willing to settle for a temporary solution
- Will benefit from a short-term gain
- Need a backup to collaboration or competition
- Feel the goals are unimportant enough to modify
- Want to make the relationship or agreement work and will settle for what is better than nothing

Some people use the compromising mode at the outset if they know they don't have the power to get what they want. You can always come back later and use another style of conflict management.

To strike a successful compromise, it is important to clarify your needs and wishes, as well as those of the other party. Then determine the areas where you agree. Once there is agreement on something, it is far easier to work out a compromise. Listening is an important part of this process. Be willing to make suggestions, and listen to what the other person says. She in turn should be willing to do the same. Be prepared to make offers, exchanges, and bargains. It is also important to identify what you are not willing to give up or budge on. The final result should be some measure of mutual satisfaction with the outcome.

Dominant and Secondary Modes

If you work only within the competitive or the avoiding mode, you limit yourself to a win-lose or a lose-lose scenario. It's natural to prefer a certain mode over others, and this one is your dominant mode. But you may also have two equally characteristic modes, such as avoiding and accommodating. This combination would indicate that you will do a lot to prevent any type of conflict. When you have two equally characteristic modes, you are *bimodal.* If you have three, you are *trimodal.*

Exhibit 5.1 should have given you an individual profile of how you respond to conflict. Now that you have read the descriptions of the five modes of managing conflict, stop and think for a moment. Which mode best describes you? Is there one that stands out, or do you feel that you use several equally? When you tallied your responses, did your profile match the way you perceive yourself?

Why Confront?

Most of the women we interviewed felt strongly that dealing with conflict and confrontation is the key to eliminating sabotage. Women need to be more supportive of other women, by being there and speaking up for them. Until women are willing and ready to confront other women on unacceptable behavior, sabotage of women by other women will continue unchecked. Nice girls may not complain, but they ought to confront.

When you know a confrontation is coming, step back and look at the dominant conflict-management style of your opponent. Your effectiveness in negotiating a resolution will be enhanced. Almost all conflicts and confrontations involve a dance, a series of moves and countermoves. Some dances end quickly; others add new movements. As you learn more about yourself and the people you work with, you will be able to act with more power and confidence. Mastering conflict and confrontation will be part of your formula.

Part Two

How to Survive and Thrive at Work

6

Speak Up and Speak Out

Nurses are learning to speak up and speak out. At hospitals in California, Massachusetts, and Texas, nurses have banded together against sexual and verbal harassment from male doctors. If any nurse sees a colleague being harassed, she calls out over the loudspeaker, "Code pink." (The phrase is based on the long-established "code blue" system that all hospitals follow when a patient is in a life-or-death emergency.) Other nurses respond by rushing to the spot and supplying support to the nurse being harassed. The nurses have learned that there is strength in numbers.

In Denver, however, when nurses in one hospital armed themselves with whistles and used them to signal "code pink," the doctors, all men, complained to the administration that if the whistleblowing didn't stop immediately, they would direct their patients to other hospitals. Financial power won and the whistles were silenced.

Venner M. Farley, dean of health professionals at Golden West College, in Huntington Beach, California, leads seminars to help nurses speak up when hospital conditions are unfair. When a physician asked her if she was one of those nursing teachers who attempt to make students think like doctors, her response was "No. Actually, I expect much more of them than that."[1]

Eliminating the Conspiracy of Silence

When respondents to the 1993 survey were asked to identify factors helping to eliminate some of the traps of the workplace, the need to speak up and speak out was the most frequent response. To be believable in any work environment, women must step away from old beliefs and eliminate the conspiracy of silence.

But women too often maintain silence, assuming that someone else will speak up for them. That's not the way the world works, however, at least not today. If you don't speak up and speak out, you are liable to be stymied by others who do. A very vocal minority ends up speaking for everyone, making decisions that affect the silent majority.

Putting Her Pen Where Her Anger Was

Sylviann Frankus is a critical-care nurse from Olympia, Washington. She is a strong believer in putting her thoughts into action. When the ABC television network premiered a new series, "Going to Extremes," Frankus was appalled by the portrayal of nurses. She fired off a letter to the network:

Dear Sir or Madam:

I'm writing in response to the remark made in the opening scenes of the first episode of "Going to Extremes." In the scene, a male medical student suggests to a female medical student that if she can't get into medical school, she might have to settle for the nursing profession. That really was a cheap shot! Nurses are nurses because they want to care for people, not because they are doctor "wannabe's."

I resent television's representation of nurses as an inferior subset of medicine. They are two separate professions. Physical therapists are not portrayed as frustrated doctors; neither should nurses be.

Does ABC realize how many nurses there are in this country? I don't think a network can afford to alienate such a large segment of its potential audience. Nurses are getting fed up with the media that just doesn't "get it." Bring us a "China Beach" rather than a "Nightingale." I have contacted the state and national nursing organizations to which I belong, to inform them of your unflattering representations of our profession.

Frankus added a postscript:

An EKG is not used for the primary diagnosis of diabetes. A fasting-glucose test would be a good idea. Perhaps you need a nurse to consult with regarding healthcare authenticity.[2]

How many other nurses would have taken the time to find out where to send such a letter, much less write it and mail it? Most of us grumble until something else comes along to replace whatever it is we were grumbling about, and most of us also assume that someone else will speak up or speak out. Many of us assume that our voices don't count. But they do. "Going to Extremes" survived only two months.

Enough Was Enough

In August 1992, I spoke at a women physicians' conference in Vail, Colorado. The other key speaker was neurosurgeon Frances Conley. The previous year, she had gone public about the sexual harassment that she had been subjected to over the years at Stanford University's medical school and hospital. She made national headlines when she resigned and spelled out her reasons in op-ed pages across the country. What Anita Hill did for corporate America, Frances Conley did for the medical community.

Reverberations echoed throughout the country. At every level of the medical community, a torrent of similar stories from women was unleashed. Conley feels that speaking out has to be viewed as a crusade to reawaken others' thinking. The need to do this is rooted in a sexist society. Conley told me about a letter she received from another woman after she went public with her statements and accusations. A portion of it read as follows:

> Men learn from early childhood that they are superior to women. They, the men, cultivate methods for keeping women in their place throughout their lives, and the behavior becomes automatic for them. Society teaches women the same thing, that men are better than we are, and we believe it.

Conley added that since women also believe that men are superior, society considers women expendable. She notes that when women hit the forty- to forty-five age bracket, they become not only expendable in the United States but also invisible.

Before meeting Conley, I had seen her on a televised panel with three other professionals: Congresswoman Pat Shroeder of Colorado; Bernadine Healey, then head of the National Institutes of Health; and a male cardiologist from New York, whose name I have repressed because I was so appalled by his remarks. The overall discussion was about earmarking of National Institutes of Health funds for research on women. The three women all supported more funds for research on women, since major health studies have usually included majority or exclusive populations of men, and few have included or been dedicated to women. The cardiologist felt that there was no reason to allocate additional funds for research on women. His rationale? "There are lots of problems that males have that have not been researched adequately, including impotence in males over sixty." His exact words were that impotence is "a huge problem for men." I just about fell off the couch laughing. My only disappointment was that the three women weren't laughing along with me.

Conley is right: women do disappear as we mature and pass through the childbearing years. Today, Conley is back at Stanford, with different rules and a great deal more respect. It wouldn't have happened if she had not chosen to speak up and speak out.

A Lollipop for a Life

By not speaking up or speaking out, we give permission for objectionable practices and behavior to continue. Lasura Gasparis Vonfrolio recalls Nurses' Week of 1992, when each of the nurses in her hospital received a lollipop with a wrapper on it that said, "You're a lifesaver":

> The CEO had been around to thank each of us, and later on the nursing supervisors gave us the lollipops. I felt insulted. The others I work with said, "Chill out. It's not a big deal. It's just a lollipop." But then I started thinking: if we had been a profession of men, or doctors, they wouldn't be handing out lollipops. I can't imagine my husband coming home from work with a lollipop and saying, "Hey, honey, look what my boss gave me!"

On Gasparis Vonfrolio's shift the night before, she had worked on a seven-year-old boy who had been hit by a car. He died, and she consoled the mother in her arms until the rest of the family arrived. There had also been a fifty-six-year old man who died of a heart attack, and a woman in her ninth month of pregnancy who had been brought into the emergency room and bled to death on her way to surgery. All in all, a routine shift. She continues her story:

I went to the CEO and told him that I do a great job, and I told him about the past twenty-four hours—that I had tried my hardest. I comforted patients and their relatives, and somehow a lollipop wouldn't do it. Something was wrong with this picture.

Then Gasparis Vonfrolio returned to the emergency room. She told the other nurses that she could accept that the CEO was ignorant; a lot of people get promoted less because of their skills than because of their politics. But what bothered her was the fact that not one of the other nurses had been willing to go with her and speak to the CEO about the inappropriateness of giving nurses lollipops:

I tried to convey to them that if all six of us had gone to talk with him, he would have heard the message and made sure that nurses were treated differently. I never found that support.

Unfortunately, when one person finally decides to break away from the pack and speak up, others usually agree that there is a problem, but few join in getting the message out. This is how the conspiracy of silence supports unacceptable behavior.

Management Doesn't Get It

Mary Ellen, a former accountant, is now a nurse manager who says her medical director is impaired by substance abuse, and the hospital will take no action:

A number of the nurses have witnessed and documented his drug and alcohol use. Nothing is ever done about it. The medical staff doesn't do an investigation, although they have the power. Their approval of the use of drugs is their nonaction.

I called my boss one day to intervene because the medical director smelled so strongly of alcohol. She did come in and confront him and then told us to mind our own business.

I've worked closely with my staff over the years to teach them techniques for dealing with conflicts. When we confront a situation that we know is dangerous, especially together, upper management consistently backs down.

We have an OB on the staff who has been here for ten years. On several occasions he has come in drunk to deliver babies and been put to bed by the nursing staff. Nothing has ever happened. This is a small community. The last few years, maternity cases are down and the hospital has hired a consultant. We have done more advertising, programs have been revamped, the facility has been redecorated, yet maternity cases continue to decline. It's not that women are having fewer babies; there are actually more. They just don't come here.

Mary Ellen is caught in a Catch-22 dilemma. Doctors do bring in revenues by their affiliations with hospitals. When they have privileges at more than one hospital, they can direct patient loads and enhance a hospital's status. Doctors are powerful.

But all that is needed to derail a hospital is a few malpractice cases. Word spreads in a community, especially a small one.

Instead of addressing the problem directly, managers hired marketing consultants to tell them how to bring in more business. If a doctor can't be detoxified, his privileges should be terminated. The nurses know this, and so do the prospective patients. Management just doesn't get it.

Send More Men

Claudia has been a staff nurse for many years. She agrees that speaking out is necessary, but she also says that if you don't follow through, speaking out doesn't work. She also believes that as more men enter nursing, nurses will move from complaining to formulating an action plan:

I've been around enough nurses to know that they complain, but they don't take an active role in the solution. I feel that when there are male nurses, it's good for us. They are inclined to say, "We have been talking about this long enough. Just do it."

Nursing schools have seen an increase in men's enrollment over the past few years, from 3 percent to 5 or 6 percent. Claudia believes that the addition of more men to the profession, coupled with a commitment to training and education in conflict resolution, will produce a new breed of nurse.

Sue Anne, a clinical educator in surgery, agrees that there is a new breed entering the profession:

My facility does a three-year diploma course. I see older staff undermining the new nurses. Many of them hold little bits of information over their heads, not giving them the full picture of a specific problem or procedure that would make it so much easier. The newer generation of nurses has learned how to ask the right questions and how to confront those who are withholding information.

Sue Anne is on the mark when she talks about education. It has to be a factor. Coupled with public awareness, it will raise the consciousness level for speaking out.

It is always nice when others speak out at the same time, but that is rare. And going solo is lonely. Friends and co-workers, who you thought were with you, mysteriously disappear and withdraw their support. By their actions, they are saying that they don't want to speak out, at least not to anyone who can make a difference.

Making Others Uncomfortable

When Gasparis Vonfrolio was called into her supervisor's office for displaying a negative attitude, her response was, "There is no such thing as a well-adjusted slave." Needless to say, her comment didn't go over well:

> My supervisor began to tell me about all the things that are wrong with me, and of course her door was open. When she was finished, all the people I work with were standing at the door and listening to her opinions about me.
>
> I could have left it at that, but I felt that her blunt remarks needed a response, especially when my co-workers had listened to every word. I told her that over the past nine years, as a nursing instructor in critical care, I had seen a lot of great nurses leave. I said there was low morale in the unit, and that the day shift was fighting with the night shift. I told her that I had seen more backstabbing in this one unit than I had seen in my whole life, and that all of it was going on under her management. I said I would work on my attitude as long as she worked on her management.

The Gasparis Vonfrolios of the world make their co-workers very uncomfortable. One reason is that when someone else speaks up and speaks out, people do agree; but because of upbringing, beliefs, and habits, it is difficult for people to express how they feel. The other person may be saying exactly what is going through their minds, but they just don't have the nerve or the skill to say it themselves. As a result, they often back away.

The Dysfunctional Workplace

As program director for the School of Nursing at the University of Colorado Health Sciences Center, Marie Miller is not surprised by the experiences of any of the women we interviewed. She strongly believes that speaking up and out is a key to resolving many problems in the workplace:

Women need to speak out sooner, instead of maintaining their silence. One of the reasons you remain silent is that you are embarrassed by what has happened. It is the same type of behavior that happens within dysfunctional families. Talking about it, even though you are embarrassed, is best. Bring it out in front, and let others discuss it with you.

Miller's recommendation to bring "it" out into the open and talk about it is an appropriate response to a dysfunctional workplace, too. There is another parallel: in a relationship that has gone sour, there comes a time when it needs to end. At work, too, if you are going to speak up and speak out, you have to be prepared to leave. As Miller says, "People have to be willing to vote with their feet."

The Media as Partners

Working with the news media is a must for the nursing profession. Interaction with the media requires monitoring, intervention, and feedback. One reporter for a major East Coast newspaper has said, "Whenever our health section carries anything about physicians that they don't like, we receive complaining phone calls immediately. Also we receive a barrage of press releases from doctors and their organizations. We never hear from the nursing organizations."[3] Another healthcare journalist stated, "With rare exceptions—the American Association of Colleges of Nursing comes to mind—major nursing organizations send us either no information at all or press releases stating only organizational positions on political or healthcare issues. We never receive any releases on innovations in nursing practice or programs, and we certainly never see anything highlighting accomplishments of individual nurses around the country or in our area. This is precisely the kind of information that is fodder for journalists."[4]

When Barbara Ruane, vice president for nursing services at East Orange General Hospital, in New Jersey, took on the popular show "Designing Women," she wrote to the producers, and then she sent a memo to all the nurses in her hospital, encouraging them to write, too. Here is an excerpt from Ruane's letter:

> A recent episode of "Designing Women," in which Julia Sugarbaker spent time in the hospital, depicted the nurse in a most negative manner. Her appearance and demeanor were offensive to the many nurses who demonstrate a professional model in their daily practice.
>
> It is curious that a show that normally portrays women in a strong and independent way would consciously choose to depict a nurse in such a demeaning way.
>
> There are over two million nurses in the United States who, every day, face life-or-death situations. They should be presented as the confident and caring professionals they are.
>
> In the future, I'm hopeful that you will depict nurses in a meaningful role.[5]

Silence = Approval

Whatever your profession is in the healthcare industry, if you don't speak up and speak out, as the women featured in this chapter have done, your silence will indicate your approval of the situation, whatever it may be. There is no way around it.

7

Compete!

Imagine that you are at work, having lunch. Your floor has been buzzing with the news that a position is opening up for a clinical specialist. You pick up your tray and join five of your colleagues, and they too have heard the news.

Amanda mentions her qualifications, and all of you agree that she is a perfect candidate. Then Sherri says that she too is planning to submit her résumé. Amanda is quiet for a moment, and then she begins to talk about the pitfalls of the position, and about courses she, Amanda, should have taken to expand her present skills. Sherri makes the same types of comments about herself.

What looked like a tense situation appears to have smoothed itself out. Everyone finishes lunch and goes back to work.

When the position is filled, neither Amanda nor Sherri gets it. Annette, another friend who was at lunch that day, gets the promotion. Hearing the other two talk about the job and the qualifications, she decided to submit her résumé.

If you were Amanda or Sherri, how would you feel? What would your reaction have been if Annette had also said she was interested in the job? You might not have been enthusiastic about someone else's putting her hat in the ring, but at least you would have known who the competition was, and you would have been able to assess her strengths and weaknesses. But the odds are quite high that your friendship with her would have been strained. Why? Among women, friends do not compete, at least not in the old-fashioned way.

In another scenario, Ellen and Patricia are two friends considering the same job. When Ellen says she is interested, Patricia may decide not to submit her résumé. Patricia may feel that it wouldn't be fair to Ellen, even if Patricia's qualifications are better. But if Ellen gets the position, Patricia may feel resentful if her friend doesn't acknowledge that one reason why she got the job is that Patricia didn't compete with her.

Competition: "Life 101"

A woman competing with other women may be blocked by old messages about being nice. There is nothing wrong with being nice while being in competition, but mixed messages may be sent and received as fear of losing surfaces: "If I'm too nice, I can't really compete. If I don't compete, I can't win. Therefore, I lose." Men are more inclined to skip being nice and to view losing as part of the school of hard knocks: that's life.

If and when you do compete with another woman, there are two unwritten rules for dealing with the outcome: whoever ends up winning should be congratulated, and then both of you must move on.

Not being the victor can give you an opportunity to do some reflecting. If you lost a promotion, did your rival have qualifications that you didn't have? If you still aspire to the promotion, are there coalitions you can form that will ease your way the next time you're at bat?

Competition is not going to go away, and there are things you can do when you are in competition. Acknowledge that competition does exist. Bring it out in the open. If a new position is available, encourage others in your group to seek it openly. If you see anyone undermining anyone else, making derogatory comments about her abilities or skills, with the intent to influence or color a decision maker's opinion, speak up and speak out. The saboteur may not be talking about you right now, but she may be in the future, when you compete with her for something.

By speaking up and confronting someone on her sabotaging behavior, you identify and open up the rules of fair play. If you win, do not gloat or act as if you are queen of the mountain. If you lose, accept your defeat. Remember, people watch those who lose as much as they watch those who win.

Missing out on an opportunity, a promotion, or an award is painful, and it's natural inclination to want to withdraw. But don't! Stay in circulation. People are going to be watching how you handle the situation.

Look First, Then Blow Your Own Horn

Phyllis, a nurse from Florida, recently applied for a supervisory position. Her approach was open competition. She let the other women she worked with know that she was applying for the job, and she even encouraged others to apply.

Not only did Phyllis land the job, she had the support of the other nurses. Word spread about her open dialogue and her encouragement of others.

But people can be suspicious, and there are times when it does not make sense to trumpet your intentions to one and all. If a position is opening up in your immediate environment, or if one is announced within the overall system of your workplace, everybody who has tapped into the grapevine is going to know, and the application process will be open to everyone.

Let's say you work at Women's Hospital, and you've heard through a friend that a position is opening up at her hospital, Good Samaritan. It sounds like your dream job. If you apply and get the job, it will not mean that you have sabotaged, undermined, or betrayed your colleagues. They may be somewhat surprised to learn that you were seeking employment somewhere else, but once they get over your impending departure, they may even ask you to keep your ears and eyes open for them. It is unlikely that you will be viewed as being in the "out group" until you leave your present position.

When you are seeking new employment outside your present organization, do not broadcast this information. After all, if you don't get the new job, your current supervisor may punish you for attempting to leave. And while you are waiting to hear whether you got the new job, management may hear about your desire to jump ship and may escort you out immediately.

From Betrayal to Shared Opportunity

Women competing with other women should "deep six" many of the messages they heard as girls. There is nothing wrong with wanting to win, and there is nothing wrong with stating your intention to go for a position, an award, or whatever is out there for you. What's wrong is the way many women have gone about it. Declare yourself and bring the rules out in the open.

If you win and get the position, that isn't a betrayal of another woman or yourself. Rather, it's an opportunity for both of you.

8

Eliminate Confrontophobia

As we have been seeing, one myth of the workplace is that nice girls do not confront. Another myth is that people who work together and are friends will not have conflicts.

Stopping the Co-conspiracy

Nice Girls Do

Donna, a nursing supervisor, had a problem with Amber, the director of advertising. Amber frequently penetrated Donna's territory and told her how she should run the office.

Donna knew she had a decision to make; Amber's meddling was irritating her more and more. Either Donna would remain quiet or she would confront Amber.

Donna decided to confront. When she did, Amber and her medical director said that if Donna did not like the way they were handling things, she could leave. Donna stepped back to evaluate the situation. After three weeks, leaving is exactly what she chose to do.

In my interview with Donna, I asked her what she would have done differently:

I'm more gutsy now, and I am more in control of myself. Usually I try to regain control of myself in an uncomfortable situation. Back then, I wasn't as knowledgeable and prepared in management issues regarding my rights as I am today.

I would have confronted her and been a little more gutsy in asking what her role and position were in confronting me, when we had both been hired by the same director. I also believe I would have ended the conversation as soon as it got going, and I would have brought in my own medical supervisor as part of the discussion. I would have told this woman to butt out.

Telling someone to butt out may bring one of two reactions: the person may be so offended by the tone of the phrase that she tunes out and doesn't hear a word you say, or she may be oblivious of that type of remark and say, "It's no big deal." In the middle of a conflict, confronting someone always takes some type of finesse. Finesse can be learned and adapted to various situations.

Role Models

Nora is director of a pediatric and young-adult short-stay surgery unit. She feels strongly that role models should be identified and techniques should be taught for dealing with conflicts and confronting people:

Women should not tolerate backstabbing and backbiting behavior. We need to have role models who will speak up and speak out. By their actions, they can demonstrate how to ease out of a conflicting situation.

I also believe we need to have team-building sessions, where inappropriate behaviors are discussed in a generic type of format. The objective is to raise others' consciousness of how destructive their behavior is and give them alternate means for dealing with it.

I feel that women in general don't like conflict and will do whatever they can to avoid it.

Is It an Age Thing?

Many people believe that women who are older are less confrontive than younger and newer players in the workplace. As an RN, Jill observes this on a daily basis:

I don't believe that women have been socialized to confront. I see changes with the newer, younger nurses in their willingness to confront. But with the older nurses, the old rules seem to be enforced. Older nurses have been socialized into nonconfrontational behavior. Women are to stay in the background and not say anything. Part of their job is to grin and bear it. When there is a problem, it is discussed among colleagues, rather than with the person it needs to be discussed with.

What Jill has described is an age-old problem that women have perfected to an art. One of my personal mottoes has become "Don't take *no* from someone who does not have the authority to say *yes*." Many times, those who need to be confronted in a situation are the yea-sayers—those who can and do make a difference when they know what the problem is. Without interacting with the person you have the conflict with, you cannot get the complete story. When you have input from the other party, you will be more effective if you need to bring in a third party or go to a higher level of authority.

Find Another Dumping Ground

As manager of a nursing staff, Louise felt that her office should not be used as a place where people could dump their problems, concerns, and opinions about others they had to work with:

As a manager, I am continually telling people to go back and discuss directly what the problem is with the person they are having it with. When they tell me they don't feel comfortable doing it, I then tell them, "Let's turn the tables. Let's say you forgot to give a patient his medication. Your colleague who followed you on the next shift comes to me with the complaint that you were irresponsible and didn't do your job. Now, how would you feel about that?" Almost always, the response is "Well, she should have come to talk to me about it first." That's when I say, "Exactly. Got to the person directly, and if it can't be resolved, then come to me."

Confronting someone means taking responsibility. It also holds the other person accountable for her actions. If you do not confront someone, your silence condones her behavior, toward you and everyone else.

Equal Pay for Equal Work

When one woman discovers that she is making less money than another who was hired at the same time or has the same title and responsibilities, it's bound to create conflict in the workplace. (And, as much as management tries to stifle information about salaries and wages, word does get out about who makes what.) Because of the "confrontophobia" that most women carry with them from childhood, a woman in this situation is most likely to do one of two things: grumble to herself (or to others who don't have the authority to do anything), or quit. Andrea, a staff development instructor, dealt with just such a problem:

Within a one-month period, there were three new hires. I was one of them. Ethel and I started in May. The third, Marta, started in June.

I felt that I was doing much more than anyone else in the office. I kept being told that because I was new, I needed to learn more. They kept giving me more and more things to do.

Ethel felt the same. We both felt overwhelmed with work.

Marta didn't seem to have the responsibilities that we did. When we went to our boss, she would say, "Marta is new, and we don't want to overwhelm her."

Months passed, but the situation didn't change. Both Ethel and I continued to be overloaded with work, but Marta was not. One day in the lunchroom, we were all talking about a variety of things, and salary came up. Marta told me what she was making, and it was more than what I was making.

I went to my boss with a practiced speech. I told her that I didn't think I was contributing less to the department than anyone else, and yet I was not paid the same, and I wondered why. I felt that I was being punished. My boss said she didn't have any control over who got paid what, and that I would have to go to her boss. That's exactly what I did. I got my raise.

Andrea did not let herself grumble about the injustice. But not enough women speak up and confront financial injustice in the workplace. By not confronting it, they give permission for it to continue.

The Boss Takes Credit

When Naomi began working at her hospital, as a clinical specialist, she learned that her supervisor was routinely taking credit for work that Naomi had produced:

My supervisor was extremely threatened when I got there. My credentials were greater than hers. In the end, a lot of the procedures that I had created and written up turned up with her name on them. I didn't feel it was worth confronting her; you have to pick your battles. I knew who had really done the work, and so did the rest of the staff.

By not doing anything, Naomi gave her boss permission to continue plagiarizing the work of others. Someone has to say, "Enough is enough." Otherwise, the thief has license to continue stealing.

Facing the Enemy

Many of us routinely confront saboteurs—but only in our imaginations. This is escapism. It's time to wake up and smell the coffee. In Chapter Five, styles of managing conflict were identified. One style is avoiding.

Avoiders make great prey for people who like to steamroll others. Women who are avoiders can be classified into three groups.

Complainers

Complainers would rather grumble, mumble, or fume about a situation. They seem to operate on the premise that everyone around them ought to be able to read their minds. When friends and coworkers ask a complainer what's wrong, her response is usually "Nothing." Women who become chronic complainers may actually enjoy being miserable and out of sync. They thrive on the attention they receive when others notice how miserable they are.

Could Have–Should Have–Ought To's

If you find yourself habitually using phrases that begin with *I could have*, *I should have*, or *I ought to*, the odds are that you are a master of avoidance. Women in this subgroup are often procrastinators. But, in their avoidance mode, they really do make decisions. They decide not to decide. If they are in an unpleasant situation, or if someone has directed undermining or sabotaging behavior toward them, they will take care of the situation in their fantasy lives. They will come up with scenarios that involve brilliant confrontations—but these never intrude on reality.

Explosives

The explosives are the ones who allow gnats to grow into elephants. When they finally erupt, often very loudly, those within hearing distance are amazed that the trigger was such a minor incident. In reality, however, an accumulation of minor incidents led to the eruption.

When the explosive finally calms down, her debris is everywhere. After a few eruptions, her apologies fall on deaf ears, and her friends and co-workers begin to distance themselves from her.

If you completed the survey in Chapter Five, then you know how to identify the dominant and backup styles that you and another person would normally use. As we saw in that chapter, there are times when it makes sense to use one style instead of another. Table 8.1 shows what works and what doesn't work in various situations. The bottom line is that most conflicts require confrontation before they can be resolved. Very few go away with no intervening action.

The Showdown

Besides recognizing your own conflict-management style, as well as that of the person with whom you are in conflict, there are a few other techniques that will enable you to move to a quicker resolution. One is to find a neutral area where you can talk with her. Your office or her office will not be ideal; each of you has her own power within her own space, and neither one can be considered neutral, nor is a public area of your workplace where others can observe and listen. Go out for

Table 8.1.   Suiting the Style to the Situation.

Style	When It Works	When It Doesn't Work
Competing	When you have the power	When others don't respect your abilities or power
Accommodating	When the other person requires status	When you need a real solution
Avoiding	When you must have the other person's participation	When you have a lot to lose When the other person is right
Collaborating	When you have time When you have a good relationship	Where there is lack of trust When time is short
Compromising	When both of you are right When you want to keep the relationship going	When only one of you is right When you have little to give

coffee, take a walk, or find a quiet place where you can sit down together.

Before the confrontation, you need to set some personal rules. First, calm down. When you are angry, step back and take a moment to compose yourself; otherwise, you'll make the best speech you will ever regret. Second, take the time to assess what has happened. Look at it from your perspective. What was the impact on you? How has it affected others? Third, take the opposite view. What do you think her perspective might be? Fourth, yawn, and then take a deep breath. You will need oxygen in your system.

A key skill is listening. As you listen, you will need to formulate any feedback you are doing to give. Tap into what your own feelings were after the conflict erupted. Be willing to acknowledge that your behavior may have been a factor in what she did, if you think that may be true.

Don't wait for the other person to come to you. Initiate the dialogue. Don't be surprised if the response is denial. If the woman you confront denies her action and her behavior, be prepared to back off. You have done what you needed to do. You have let her know that her behavior, what you experienced and observed, was not okay. If she is responsible for her behavior, she probably knows it. There are exceptions, but few people are in total denial or completely cut off from the real world.

After you confront her, drop it. Move on, and go about your business. This does not mean that you are to be all-forgiving. The new factor in the equation is that now you are alert. You are aware that her objectionable behavior did occur, and that you confronted her. Now you need to keep a watchful eye open for recurrences. If there are any, you immediately confront her again.

It will probably take a few confrontations for her to stop doing whatever she is doing to you or to others. Confronting is rarely easy, but it will be less stressful for you every time you do it; after all, you are learning a new behavior, too. At some point, she should realize what her actions and activities are doing to you and to others.

Talking with another person face-to-face is usually the best way to confront her. That way, she can see your body language, and you can see hers. You can observe whether she is listening. Face-to-face confrontations do require you to be coolheaded and to have your facts together. Otherwise, emotions may cause you to go on the attack, which only makes matters worse.

If it is impossible to have a face-to-face encounter, writing is probably your second-best choice. You may not know whether she has actually read what you've written, but writing does give you the opportunity to set out the facts as you understand them and let her know what the impact of her behavior has been. Before you send a letter, have a trusted confidante read it to eliminate any inappropriate sharpness or overemotional remarks. This is a time for "just the facts," as you perceive them. Writing also gives you the luxury of time, but that can be a disadvantage: if you wait too long to confront her, she may not have a clue about what she did or why you are upset.

Another way to confront someone is over the phone, but this choice has several disadvantages. First of all, 55 percent of communication comes through gestures and body language, and 38 percent comes from tone. Words carry only 7 percent of the message. This means that 93 percent of what you say is actually unspoken. Second, when you confront someone by phone, you can't be sure she is listening. She can put you on hold, walk away, or even hang up before you are aware the call has been disconnected. And even if you do both remain on the line, you can't see her face, her eyes, or her body language, nor can she see yours, your anger, or your hurt. That happens only when she is physically in your space.

Whenever you realize that you have been undermined, backstabbed, or held up to ridicule by anyone you work with or thought was your friend, you must confront. Your opening line can be something like this: "It's been brought to my attention that you have been saying negative things about me behind my back. If that's true, I want you to know that I am offended, and I want it to stop."

9

Identify and Circulate the Unwritten Rules

One year, I spoke at the annual convention of a healthcare group. I usually bring copies of my books and audiotapes for participants to purchase if they so choose. Our policy has never been to pitch them; rather, they are available if anyone is interested. If no one wants to buy any, it's not a big deal. They are packed up and returned to my office in Denver. When we do make a sale, we also make a donation to a particular cause or fund that the sponsoring group has identified, and we base the donation on a percentage of sales. Alternatively, we offer books and tapes, worth several hundred dollars, for the group's library. The group states its choice. My right to make books, tapes, and videos available is a provision included in my standard contract.

There were several workshops going on at the same time as mine. The woman who had hired me was checking in on each one, to see how things were going. When she got to mine, she wasn't happy. In fact, she was very angry. The reason for her anger was a table displaying books and audiotapes. She could barely control her wrath. She said they had to be immediately boxed up and put away. Her unwritten rule was that no products could be sold. At break time, everything was boxed up and put out of sight.

Since I was in the first quarter of an all-day workshop, I thought this would be a great example to use when I got to the section on unwritten rules. I told her I wasn't psychic. It was normal to have support tools—books and tapes—available, and this had not been excluded from our contract. My words were meaningless to her. I had violated her unwritten rule, and she forbade me to use it as an example in the workshop. She also forbade my giving any books away, which I normally do during certain activities in a program that involves audience participation.

In retrospect, I regret that I did not use her unwritten rule as an example. The situation was extremely unfortunate, but I learned a lesson: I now make sure that when I talk with the people in charge they really understand what is in my contract, and I ask what the specific rules are, if any, for their presenters.

When unwritten rules are not communicated, a lose-lose situation is created. In my situation, we had three identifiable losers: the participants, who were angry because they could not purchase the books and tapes; the association, because this woman created a great deal of ill will among the participants; and myself, since I had the hassle of shipping items that were not used, the disruption of boxing them up, irritation that her rule had not been explained to me, and the possibility that my performance would be affected by her negativism and her way of announcing her unwritten rule. How much easier it would have been for all of us if the unwritten rule had been revealed before I was required to live and work by it.

Discovering the Unwritten Rules

The first time I conducted a workshop on sabotage in the healthcare workplace, I divided participants into different groups for a series of exercises. One of the exercises was to brainstorm in small groups of three to six individuals, in order to identify various unwritten rules in the workplace. I told them, "There are two identifiable rules in the workplace: go to work, and do the job. It's the four hundred unwritten rules that can destroy your working relationships and your work environment." Then I gave an example of an unwritten rule: in the coffee room, the first person in makes the first pot, and the person who takes the last cup of coffee makes a new pot. I gave another example: in the copy room, if someone switches from regular to legal-size paper, she is supposed to switch back to regular for the next person; if someone uses fuchsia paper for a flyer, the unwritten rule is to switch back to white.

These rules seem commonsensical, but when these kinds of unwritten rules are not followed, they seed discontent. A single incident may not seem important, but over a period of time, many small infractions can make life a monstrous hassle.

Unwritten rules that participants in our workshops have identified include the following:

Bosses

- Showcase the boss.
- Don't bug the boss when his or her door is closed.
- Avoid the boss when he or she is in a bad mood.
- The boss can do whatever he or she wants.
- Bosses are responsible for being happy and solving problems.
- In meetings, your opinions should follow the leader's (don't rock the boat).

Managers

- Managers work on their days off.
- Managers can fix things on short notice.
- Managers are on duty twenty-four hours a day.

- Managers always know what's right.
- White males are in charge.
- Women do not hold top-level executive positions.
- Managers don't take days off close to a deadline.
- Managers don't take two weeks of vacation time in a row.
- Managers don't call in sick to a hospital on holidays or weekends.

Nurses

- Nurses are on duty twenty-four hours.
- Nurses should be willing to do anything.
- The best nurses take the worst assignments.
- The best nurses do things no one else will.
- Nurses always respond immediately.
- Full-timers should have more influence.
- Nurses should not take responsibility for peers; they should grumble instead.
- Whoever is stuck with the narcotic keys has to do the report.
- Never take pens out of the nursing office.
- The previous shift doesn't have to complete its work.
- If there is a mistake, blame it on the student.
- If there is a mistake, blame it on the new nurse.
- Nurses with false fingernails cannot do patient care.
- Don't call male doctors by their first names.
- Never call a resident between 7 A.M. and 8 A.M.
- Call residents by their first names, but with patients, call them "Doctor."

- Doctors can do anything.
- Don't undermine the doctor; she or he has the final say.
- Doctors are always right.
- Call women doctors by their first names.
- Don't sit in the doctor's chair.
- Always make rounds with doctors.
- Drop everything when the doctor enters.
- Doctors' wives get special treatment.

Teams

- Support all decisions of the team, even if you disagree.
- Act professionally at all costs.
- Bring out the best in other team members.
- Develop departmental loyalty.
- Cover for each other.
- Don't air the team's dirty laundry.
- Help another team member when your work is completed.
- Follow the chain of command.
- Don't brag.
- Be supportive.
- Give credit where it is due.
- Don't be a martyr; if you are busy, ask for help.
- Everyone should pitch in.
- If you come last, you lose.
- Whoever enters the last recording starts a new sheet.
- Let people know where you are.

- Look busy even if you are not.
- Part-time people can't refuse assignments.
- If it's not documented, you did not do it.
- Doing extra work is brown-nosing.
- Cover your ass.

The Work Environment

- No handwritten signs.
- No tape on doors.
- Fill the soap dispenser.
- First one in turns on the copier.
- Return the copy machine to the regular setting if you change it.
- If the copier is empty, fill it.
- If you use it, put it back the way it was.
- Keep areas neat.
- Return all dishes to the kitchen, and wash the ones you use.
- The secretary makes the coffee.
- No one can drink coffee if the supervisor is present.
- Don't use someone else's coffee cup.
- Get a cup of coffee before you answer any questions.
- If it's broken, fix it.
- Reset the postage meter.
- Don't unplug equipment.
- First one in turns the lights on; last one out turns them off.
- Clean up after yourself.
- Don't sit on the counters.

- Don't read newspapers or magazines at your desk.
- Office property is everyone's; treat it so.
- Whoever stuffs it empties it.
- Don't sit in someone's favorite chair.
- Don't touch someone's computer without permission.
- No gifts on birthdays; cakes only.
- If you smoke, pick up your cigarette butts.

Co-workers

- Smokers can take more breaks than nonsmokers and get away with it.
- Smokers regularly take all breaks and lunches.
- Night shifts don't take breaks.
- Too many bathroom breaks are frowned on.
- Certain people get specific time slots for lunch and dinner.
- Parents can be on the phone more than nonparents.
- Parents get certain holidays off.
- Parents don't have to work overtime.
- Parents can take time off.
- Parents can take more sick days off.
- When their kids are selling candy, calendars, and cookies, parents can pressure you to buy them.

Miscellaneous Unwritten Rules

- Friday is dress-down day.
- Maintain a proper personal appearance.
- Don't wear jeans.

- Managers don't wear striped ties.
- It's not the money that counts; you work to take care of others.
- If you don't take assigned work, you will get your hours cut back.
- If you do the work of a charge nurse, don't assume you will get paid as one.
- You don't get paid if you work overtime.
- If you cared, you would work more.
- Keep messages.
- Return calls promptly.
- Answer the phone by the second ring.
- Personal calls are to be brief.
- Volunteer to keep notes.
- If you understand the form, it is time to change it.
- Always eat with the same people, or suffer.
- Tell someone she has lipstick on her cheek or teeth.
- Learn the "old boy" rules.
- If you take a risk, you had better be right.
- Tell me; do not surprise me.
- Do it the way it's always been done.
- Always act like a lady.
- If you volunteer, you will get picked on.
- It's not what you do, it's whom you know.
- Smile even if you don't like it.
- If you speak out, you are a complainer.
- You get feedback only when you grumble.

- Don't be happy or else someone will squash you.
- Give visitors directions.
- You cannot turn down a patient's request.

What Unwritten Rules Do You Work Under?

Set aside fifteen to thirty minutes over the next few days, and just ponder scenarios in your workplace. Identify the different individuals you work with, those in management or supervisory positions and those in senior management, including your CEO. Next, list the women and men you work with directly.

As you identify the women and men in your workplace, describe their tasks, their personalities, and the interactions you have with them. Ask yourself if they dress or speak in specific ways. Have the times when you had direct interaction with them been good, bad, or indifferent? Is your workplace stimulating and energetic, or is it a drag for you to show up each day?

Write down your thoughts about the various individuals you work with. When images of your boss, supervisor, or manager come to mind, are there any idiosyncrasies, mandates, or dicta that also come to mind?

Now think about your colleagues and co-workers. Do you have rules regarding days off, break time, interactions, or housekeeping? No matter how minor they seem, write these rules down. Violation of unwritten rules can drive others crazy. If you or someone else continually violates or ignores them, enormous friction is created.

Next, brainstorm with a trusted colleague to expand your list, or at least collaborate on one. In staff meetings, if there is time set aside for comments and questions, you can involve others in identifying various unwritten rules.

If your manager or supervisor is not open to this idea, she may perceive your suggestion as threatening. If so, or if you are unsure about how your manager will respond, it may be better to approach your manager on a one-to-one basis. Since your objective is to identify unwritten rules and make life in your workplace more livable, try saying something like this: "Since I've been here, I have noticed a series of things that many of my co-workers do." Next, identify some of those things. It could be that everyone washes her own coffee cup, that certain coffee cups are not used, and that smoking is allowed only in certain areas. Everything you mention should be basically safe and nonthreatening. Continue with a statement like this: "If I had known that these were unwritten rules, it would have been so much easier for me when I started here. Has anyone thought about putting together a notebook of other rules that our team goes by? When we add new employees or have temps and floaters, this could give them a better understanding of what makes our unit tick."

A manager who declines to identify your team's unwritten rules, or who is insensitive to the need to do so, will be the exception. Encourage her to bring the topic up at a meeting, and reaffirm that if you had known some of the rules when you first arrived, you could have been more effective and efficient in your job.

Sometimes remaining anonymous is important, for personal or even political reasons, and a suggestion-type box can be used to collect the unwritten rules. And some of the rules that emerge will be absurd, sacred cows that everyone knows about and dislikes but that still are untouchable.

Rules Change

Before assuming that an unwritten rule really is untouchable or unchangeable, ask why? If you are not sure, ask someone you work with. Sometimes no one really knows why some rules are in place. Identify those rules and talk about them, and maybe they can be changed. (The group may also decide to keep them, of course.)

Above all, have some fun identifying the unwritten rules of your workplace. Why not post an Unwritten Rule of the Week and have a good laugh with your co-workers?

Breaking the Unwritten Rules

The following case histories tell how women have been sabotaged because they did not know the unwritten rules of their workplace.

Learning the Ropes

Jill loves her patients, and she loves nursing. She also feels she would be better off if she could work in a vacuum because she has seen so many miserable things that established nurses have done to new nurses. She feels strongly that established nurses should open up during orientation so that new nurses will understand all the nuances of what is expected of them:

> The older nurses expect a lot more of the newer nurses. They are brand new and are going to make mistakes. Why they expect them to know all the rules, all the requirements, and all the personalities of the other nurses on the floor is beyond me. There is a lot of bitching going on, and there are times I do not know why I do what I do. I love nursing. I just wish the atmosphere was more collaborative.

Lunchtime Is Not Personal Time

Holly is a health-unit coordinator with a large hospital in Montana, working in a nonemergency sector of the hospital. She recalls a time when she decided to take care of some of her personal business during her lunch hour. Unfortunately, in Holly's workplace there were unwritten rules dealing with just how far she could wander during her lunch hour:

I left the hospital premises to pay a bill. Later, I was informed that it was an infringement of hospital policy to leave the premises during my shift.

Dorian, who would normally cover my desk during lunch, had called down to say that her partner, Felicia, was leaving early because she was ill. Therefore, the two of us should go to lunch now, while Felicia was still there, so she could leave when we got back.

This did not make sense to me, since we could stagger our leaving times. I told her to go ahead and go, and I would go to lunch later because I had to pay a bill in the village. Dorian is not well liked within the hospital. She has a reputation for being bossy, and she likes to run things. I waited to go to lunch until she came back and offered to cover for Felicia so she could go home.

Our boss happened to call in, and Dorian told her that I was going to leave the premises to pay a bill. A few days later, I was called into her office and was reprimanded for violating hospital policy. When I responded that I did not know it wasn't allowed and was against the rules, I received no support. I've been with the hospital for fifteen years.

Holly was in a situation where a co-worker did not like her independence, and she was angry that Holly didn't do what she wanted her to do—take lunch now. Holly wasn't aware of any policy that would have forbidden her to go the six blocks to pay her bill. Later, when Holly went to her boss's boss to inquire about the rule, she was told only that employees had to stay in close proximity to the hospital.

People can be very myopic and close-minded. They see only black and white, never shades of gray. It is understandable to ask someone in a critical-care unit or an emergency room to stay within a very short distance of the work station during breaks and lunch hours. Holly was a clerk. She was someone who would not have been involved in a life-or-death situation.

Until the rule changes, Holly will stay close to work on all breaks. For practical purposes, it would make sense for her employer to re-address and update this rule. After all, hospitals are about getting and staying well. Taking a walk is certainly healthier than sitting in a room or out on a bench.

Not in My Department

Sharon is director of surgical services with a hospital that is very family-oriented in terms of patients and employees alike. She re-members the time she fired two nurses. When the CEO found out, she was very upset. She told Sharon that she should have found a way to keep them, no matter what. The unwritten rule was that you didn't fire anyone.

Once employees understand that a rule like "We do not fire anyone" exists, that rule can lower morale and innovativeness and prevent the learning of new things. It can even encourage goofing off. It's like a disease that no one wants to talk about. Rather, people keep quiet, failing to recognize that such a rule can poison the whole work environment:

> I knew the hospital rule that you did not fire someone. I asked another department head to take them on her staff, and she told me that she did not want to. I knew I wasn't going to keep them on my staff, so I had no choice. Now I am viewed as a coldhearted bitch. In my professional opinion, they were a liability to me, as well as to the patients I serve.

Unwritten rules that say "Do anything to retain personnel" cre-ate enormous problems. Many times, the person who is retained will be an older employee, one who is close to retirement. She may be slowing down or her skills may be substandard and outmoded. Management believes that because she has been with the establishment for so many years, she should be rewarded for her dedication and loyalty. The unwritten rule is that management owes this to the employee. But is that true? When someone is not required to maintain a level of continuing education and competence, such laxity can lead to mediocrity and even danger. Sharon had this problem in another instance, too:

> I recently had another serious breach of discipline, due to negligence. I believed that two more nurses should be fired. We had done a case in surgery where the instruments had not been sterilized. When I questioned the nurses, they said that they knew what they were supposed to do, but they just didn't do it. They never gave me a reason why. Because of the culture of the hospital, I couldn't fire them. I had to pass their mediocrity on to some other department and hold my breath that a lawsuit does not hit.
>
> I think that dedication and loyalty mean so much here that people who are problems are held on to and put into places where they cannot cause as many problems as before. At least, that's the theory.
>
> After I fired the first two nurses, there was a big meeting. It was the first time anyone had ever been fired from the operating-room staff. Everyone was shocked. At the meeting, the CEO said she hated getting up in the morning and coming to work when the staff was not happy to be working. I felt that her remarks were very inappropriate. After all, she can't be responsible for the staff's happiness.

Sharon is correct. People may be unhappy or happy for a variety of reasons, many of which may have nothing to do with the workplace. What the boss should be responsible for is creating an environment that is safe, meets various standards, delivers what it promises, and rewards competence.

Mandating Rules All

Natalie is a nurse who has one child and is expecting another. In her hospital, if the following shift looks shorthanded, the nurse manager can mandate someone to work a second shift. Usually the person mandated to work is the low woman on the totem pole:

> Normally, I work a three-to-eleven shift three days a week. I came on as an extra one day and was scheduled to work that shift. When the charge nurse said she was going to mandate me to work the next shift, eleven-to-seven, I told her that she could not do that, since I had agreed to work as an extra. She should then have gone and found the next appropriate person to work the night shift. But that person turned out to be a single parent with two kids. Because of that, the charge nurse volunteered to do the extra shift herself.

Natalie brings up a very sensitive point: she is married, and the other woman is not, but both women are mothers. Just because someone is married, management should not assume that a spouse is available for child care. Natalie works the evening shift, and the assumption is that her spouse works the day shift; that should leave her available to fill in on the night shift, because her husband could be with their child:

> If the single mother had been mandated, she would have had two shifts and then had the responsibility for her child—but so would I. My experience with the unwritten rules is that single mothers get more understanding, leeway, and preference.

Natalie mentioned another unwritten rule. She is certified in chemotherapy, and the unwritten rule is that if you are so certified, you have to take on assignments. The exception is that if you are pregnant and in your first trimester, you do not have to do chemotherapy. During the time when Natalie was trying to get pregnant, there was a two-week period of uncertainty each month, until her pregnancy was confirmed:

> We were going through a staff shortage and had a bunch of open holes. If you knew chemo, you had to do it, even if you didn't want to or said no. If I had said no without a confirmed pregnancy, I could have been fired. Eventually, I transferred off the floor.

Use Your Head

Kim is a staff doctor in the emergency room of a medium-size hospital in the South. She says she did not realize how bright she was until she was in her thirties. That's when she decided to stop being a nurse and enroll in medical school. Kim feels that one unwritten rule should be "Use your head." She has been with her present hospital for two years and finds that it is difficult to get rid of the old unwritten rules and let common sense prevail:

> Sometimes I get aggravated with the nurses. We can have a waiting room full of people, and in comes a twenty-six-year-old man who says he has chest pains, and they move a child with a temperature of 105 degrees to the back burner. The young man has waited three weeks to come in, and here we have a child with a high fever. It irritates the hell out of me.
>
> The nurses should have enough sense to make these decisions. I know that nurses have brains in their heads. I was a great nurse, and so were most that worked around me. When I questioned their judgment about bringing in the young man with chest pains first, they said, "Well, he was here first." My response to that was "This is not a damned bakery."

Several times I have made a general statement about the waiting room: children with high temperatures are seen first. My policy is not to let these children wait for three hours. I have found that if I go individually to the nurses and restate my policies, they feel that they are being singled out and discriminated against.

My style is to be more blunt, but I have found that I have to change and be more subtle. If I don't, I could have a situation where somebody who is sixty years old, blue in the face, vomiting, and having massive chest pain will be held back while they bring in a child with a 102-degree temperature. It seems absurd, but that's what happens. My rule is to use your head.

Circulating the Unwritten Rules

Every workplace has unwritten rules, and they are different in each one. Some may need to be changed. They all need to be communicated, passed along from those who know them to those who don't.

As you learn the unwritten rules, speak up. You need to pass them along to others. When you are oblivious of the unwritten rules, or when you don't speak out and pass them along, you set yourself up for a fall. You set others up, too, and everyone loses.

10

Develop and Expand Teams

If you were to gather a group of managers from a variety of industries and organizations and ask them to identify the top three elements of creating an effective workplace for all—management, employees, and customers—being a team player and participating in teamwork would be on everyone's list. Team play, teamwork, and team members are interchanged continually in your workplace. Some teams have one member in one location; others have many members in numerous locations.

For many, the phrase *team player* almost has a tainted air about it. In the past, being a team player meant keeping your mouth shut, working long hours, and not speaking up when someone else took the credit. But today's work teams don't need to use sports metaphors to interact with each other. They do, however, need to understand that each member of the team has the potential to be a key player, no matter the size and number of locations of the team. Michelle Jackman describes a key player in her excellent book *Star Teams, Key Players*: "A Key Player is a peak performer plus. She can be found in any job at any level of the organization. She does her job with consistent excellence, but she's also acquired a second set of skills—team skills—that make her an indispensable member of her team. Because her unique combination of skills can't be easily replaced, she has more leverage, is presented with more opportunities and choices, and has greater latitude in shaping her own career than her peers in the workplace."[1]

As the healthcare industry evolves, teams will be a critical element—not just people coming together to work on a project or a report, but teams made up of key players, the star teams of the next millennium. Jackman describes the team of the future: "A Star Team accomplishes its tasks with a high degree of energy, harmony and enthusiasm. It repays the effort of individual members by protecting and nurturing their careers and providing them with challenge, responsibility, opportunity, and—above all—recognition for their labors."[2] The new-style team will win more than it loses. It will focus on getting results, not just on personalities, processes, and rules. In the workplaces, it will tap talent, time, and energy to get things done. Games, politics, and grandstanding don't belong, nor do they fit.

For any team to succeed, all the players must have a common vision and the desire to succeed at their goal. Players must complement each other, recognizing that not everyone has the same strengths and weaknesses, and being prepared to compensate for or offset others' weaknesses.

Imagine that you are a new member of a team. It looks as if civil war could break out at any time. The key problem is that conflicts can't be resolved, and members are being pulled into opposing factions. Several problems have come to your attention:

- When one coalition or faction makes a successful presentation, the other reacts with hurt feelings.

- When ideas are brainstormed and offered, team conflict erupts, and members are told to forget what they are working on.

- When work is completed, members bury it, not telling the leaders that the project is done.

- New members of the team quickly learn that they have to align themselves with one of the factions.

- One of the team's co-leaders is angry because her protégé or mentor doesn't receive respect from everyone.

Sound familiar? This could be your company, hospital, or association. It could even be your family. No matter how successful a product, company, or organization is, a divided team is costly. Energy, money, talent, and time disappear into a black hole. Team warfare is crazy. It's destructive, stressful, and unproductive. Leaders and players must step back and assess their teams.

Phases of Team Development

Cohesive teams aren't created overnight. As a team develops, it evolves through phases. Teams in the first phase are usually individual-centered, with each participant having separate goals rather than group ones. Individuals have no responsibility for others, tend to avoid change, and are not willing to deal with conflict. As the members get to know each other, new purposes and responsibilities are defined, the skills of various members are identified, and communication expands.

The second phase is more developmental. Individuals identify with the group. Purposes are clarified and expanded. Roles and various norms for working together are established. In this phase, a team tends to be leader-centered. The leader provides direction, assigns tasks, and evaluates performance. She is usually at the center of all communication.

In the third and final phase, the team is purpose-centered, and the members understand and use the purpose to guide action and decisions for the team as a whole. (An excellent resource for team building is Steven Buchholz's *Creating the High-Performance Team*.)

Every team has problems. What happens when you are involved with a team and it just doesn't get off the dime, or when certain members don't carry their share of the load and others seem to dominate? On any team, whether newly formed or established, there will be breakdowns in communication, tasks, and cohesion. As a participant or a team leader, it's important for you to recognize problems when they are just beginning. Common problems include fragmentation, lack of productivity, lack of motivation, resentment, misbehavior, dominating and submissive personalities, overdependence on the leader, too much accommodation and too little challenging, lack of interest, and failure to deal with conflict. These are all problems that will surface at various times throughout the evolution of any team. As a leader or as a member, you must not ignore any problem. Avoidance should be squashed. Arriving at the third phase of team development involves hard work. The adage "Anything worthwhile is worth working for" applies.

Women on Teams

After a merger, when staffs are combined and people are let go, problems often surface. Not everyone knows everyone else, protection of turf increases, and trust among co-workers has not yet developed. These phenomena are all normal whenever there are "new kids on the block." In the changing context of the healthcare industry, issues like these will be more and more common, as we'll see in the following case histories.

Here Today, Gone Tomorrow

Georgia, a staff RN, works in a hospital that merged with another. Her manager was let go, and the manager from the other hospital was retained.

Georgia reports that her floor is very busy. Normally, the nursing staff was sufficient to cover needs and emergencies, but ever since the merger there has been more pressure on all the nurses. Georgia's previous nurse manager had gone out of her way to help and fill in, as necessary; an unwritten rule was that team members should offer that kind of support. But now, Georgia says, things have changed.

> I don't understand it. When we get busy and need help, she is gone. Since she has been here, it's happened three out of five days. It's awful.

Overstepping Boundaries

Marilyn is the head nurse of an intensive-care unit. During the process of selecting a new director of nursing, Marilyn and two others ran the department until the position was filled.

The new nursing director didn't last long: she was fired after six months. Whatever got in her path ended up damaged, and it took more than six months to put the teams back together after she left:

> The new director of nursing strongly believed in having people who were educated differently from the way I had been. She would place large, unacceptable expectations on people. It was virtually impossible to complete the tasks that she would assign. She constantly picked at you, and there was nothing that anyone did that was right, even though three of us had been functioning in her role for the past six months. Within six months, everyone had put in for a transfer. They just couldn't take it any longer.
>
> She was very aggressive and very demanding. There was no attempt to collaborate or get input from any of us. I believe that one of the factors in letting her go was that she overstepped the small-town atmosphere that our hospital had.

Fear Fills the Air

As a relief nursing supervisor, Cam sees factions everywhere. Mergers, hiring freezes, and layoffs have all had a substantial impact on the hospital where she works. With healthcare's changing marketplace, fear seeps out of every corner. When there is fear, it's difficult to work effectively as a team member or as a team leader. In her work role, Cam has been able to observe firsthand the chaos and confusion of the past year:

> I think hospitals are having a very difficult time. Administration is getting pressure from physicians, nursing staff, and the general public. It's as though everybody is against everybody else. The insurance companies are in one corner, administration is in another, physicians are in another, and the nurses are in another. Around the corner is the union, and then there is the general public.
>
> Everyone seems to want their own power, and factions position themselves with the belief that their way is best. Nobody wants to work together. It's like we have a bunch of special-interest groups.

What Cam is reporting is quite common in hospitals today. A common remark I heard among the women interviewed was that centralized communication is lacking.

It is impossible to build a team—whether it is a small unit, a floor, or the entire hospital—unless there is communication. Two factions that Cam did not name are the government and lawyers. Each is a major contributor to the fear that permeates the hospital environment.

Hospitals Can't Be Assembly Lines

When change is in the air, the old rules often do not work. To create and build on new rules, people have to talk. Many hospitals today try to run their operations with an assembly-line or cookie-cutter approach when it comes to patient care. But patients come in all shapes, sizes, and colors. Some need a lot more care and attention than others.

In Natalie's hospital, however, the administration has developed a formula for patient loads:

> Our hospital runs like an assembly line. We have HPPD—hours per patient day. It doesn't matter how acutely ill our patients are. They staff our floor with a graph. If it's the day shift, and there are thirty patients, you get so many nurses. In the afternoon and night shifts, you may have the same patient load, with the same number of acutely ill patients, but now you get fewer nurses. That's because of the assumption that most people sleep more during the night.
>
> On my floor, on any given day, there will be seven patients with leukemia. Leukemia patients take a lot of time. They may have just finished chemo, their counts have dropped, and they are continually given blood or blood products. Three leukemia patients could need the attention and care that ten others might need.

A Reluctant Leader

Jill says that her new nurse manager doesn't like disciplining the nurses. She wants the nurses to work out their problems among themselves:

> She is very open to suggestions, but she pretty much steps back from the management role as far as the nurses on the floor are concerned. She manages the floor with the daily activities of the unit. When it comes to managing the nursing, that's in our own hands. We have self-governance on our floor, so all the nurses do their own scheduling.

Closing the Ranks

As a nursing assistant, Sally feels that team efforts in healthcare are essential. But her observation is that few practice teamwork. If people did, the work load would be less overwhelming:

> I feel we really have to talk to one another; it's a team effort. Some of the nurses don't realize that. When I'm working with an RN, I feel that part of my job is to tell her about any unusual things I notice about the patients. There are several nurses on my floor who act as though they are above everything. I know I'm not an RN. But when you work closely with patients—whether it's bathing them, changing their bed linens, or helping them up— you tend to notice things that may not be apparent to nurses when they pass out the medication.

What Sally is experiencing is a form of professional snobbery.

Getting the Best

Kendall was surprised to be hired as director of a successful women's health center in California. The hospital that she works for is religiously affiliated. Mary, the vice president, had shaped the hospital's vision and had responsibility for expanding various services. She is a Catholic, and so her religious beliefs accord with the hospital's philosophy. But Kendall feels that Mary has made a point of hiring the best people, regardless of faith:

> I don't know if Mary said out loud, "I'm going to bring in non-Catholics." What she did say was that she was going to bring in the right person for the right job. Today, our six directors are not all Catholics; they are half and half. When Mary first came on board, she got rid of a lot of people. Some were let go. Others were moved into other positions. It was actually done quite smoothly, over a period of time.

Mary had a vision of what she wanted her team to look like. The six directors under her meet on a weekly basis to share what's going on. We really do work as a team. Because of Mary's efforts to involve all the major players in the hospital on an ongoing basis, we are aware of what's happening in other areas and can give intelligent answers when asked about the workings of the hospital.

In many ways, Kendall's setting is ideal. Planning is an important element of effective team development, and Kendall says that before anyone is hired, she or he undergoes several days of testing, to see whether there is a good fit with the environment and with the teams that are so much a part of this organization.

Breaking the Silence

If there is harmony in a workplace, and if a team is working effectively, members are more inclined to speak up when something is out of sync. Lorraine is a director of women's and children's services. She recalls two instances when women in her group were up for promotion but got passed over:

The people who were conducting tenure reviews didn't have enough information about the contributions of these women. In one particular instance, several of us put together a meeting to review the situation.

The meeting was not made up of people who were administrators and had power, but we did invite those individuals to join us. All of us wrote letters about what was happening and about how this woman was passed over. She eventually got her promotion and is now dean of the school of nursing.

Here was a group that rose to support one of its members, who had been overlooked. There may have been people in the group who wanted the promotion themselves, but the group's sense of fairness prevailed.

Who Was Here First?

When Gaye was promoted to head nurse, she had to lay off a member of her staff, and a little team support would have made a big difference:

> Never in the history of the hospital had we let anyone go. My supervisor told me that the layoff would be by seniority and would be done in a month.
>
> When I had my staff meeting, I told the nurses that there would be a layoff in a month, based on seniority. They all asked who it would be. Without my naming names, they figured it out: Juanita.
>
> Juanita was very upset. I didn't want to lose her. I felt that she was very valuable, and I told her so.
>
> The atmosphere on our floor had a heavy cloud over it. I sharpened my pencil and started to move the nurses' hours around. With these manipulations, I estimated that if everyone would reduce her hours by four hours per month, I could retain Juanita's position. I felt very good about finding a solution.
>
> Then it turned out that the person to be laid off was not Juanita. It was Cheryl, who had been hired a week later. The next week, I called a meeting and put out my proposal to reduce everyone's hours and save the position. Juanita was the one who would not give up four hours to save her co-worker's job! And she ended up filing a complaint with the union.

If We Disagree . . . You're Still O.K.

Change brings fear. When it happens to you, it's scary and intimidating. When you are an active participant, change can be exciting and exhilarating. Mary Ellen, the nurse manager of a mental health unit, is attempting to bring some of that excitement into the team-building programs she has implemented:

> We are doing team building throughout our whole unit. Communication skills are being taught. People are being shown methods for confronting conflict. We are really looking at a phenomenon that women seem to get stuck with: "If I disagree with you, then you are a bad person, and I won't like you anymore."
>
> With all the information we have about communicating, you'd think we would be skilled at it in our unit. But we get stuck, just like everyone else. Our next phase is to look at our various roles—what our expectations are of each other, and whether those expectations are realistic.

Initially, Mary Ellen met a great deal of resistance. It has taken her over a year to get the attention of the members of her team. All of a sudden, though, they are starting to move quickly, saying that things are better than they've ever been.

Mary Ellen feels that, overall, progress has been excellent. Her unit had been notorious for its problematic staff. They had major crises, didn't know how to behave at work, and reacted negatively to the most minor events. The change speaks well for Mary Ellen's leadership. She hasn't given up hope even during rough, nonresponsive periods with the staff. She has held to her vision and is beginning to see the rewards.

Enjoyment Isn't in the Job Description

As an emergency-room physician, Kim has found a great deal of support from her male colleagues. She recalls a few occasions when nurses in the emergency room complained to administrators that they did not "enjoy" working with her. The complaints had led to Kim's being dropped from the duty roster:

> It was the male physicians who called major meetings and dragged the administrators into them. The men would say, "What the hell do you think you're doing? She is one of the best doctors we have ever had in the emergency room. We don't really give a damn if Nurse So-and-So does not enjoy working with her just because Kim tells her how she wants certain things done."

Kim, you will recall, is the doctor who had problems with the emergency-room nurses when they treated a young man with chest pains and left a child in the waiting room with a 105-degree temperature. Kim confronted the nurses, and their complaints to a third party are not surprising. The "get even" response is common. Kim does have the support of her male colleagues, but it would be better if she had the support of women on the staff—the people she spends far more time with.

Respect Is the Magic Word

Peggy's experiences have been better than Kim's. Peggy is a partner in a family practice in Connecticut, and she says that her tail has been saved by good nurses over the years. Her way of working with nurses starts from respect:

> The male interns, residents, and doctors tend to hand down orders. I think some of the women doctors tend to do the same thing because they get into competition with the nurses.
>
> I've been on the receiving end of that. Nurses have a problem accepting orders from me, but not from the male interns. They then look at me as if to say, "I can do this as well as you." It's a form of competition. I try to defuse the situation by actively working with them. Any doctor who doesn't respect the experience and value of the nurses loses out.

Respect, besides being Peggy's magic word, is a key factor in building an effective team.

An "Abnormal" Teacher

As an instructor at the College of Staten Island, Laura Gasparis Vonfrolio discovered that some of her nursing students didn't do well on tests, even when they knew the material. Her solution was unique:

> When you take a test, you want to get the best grade. I found that there are students who do not do well, for a number of reasons. It may be that they don't study, but there are times when they just freeze up.
>
> My solution was to take the students who got B's or C's and pair them with the students who got A's. The role of the A student was to work with the B or C students and make that student get an A. Once that happened, all my A students were exempt from any other exams. It almost always worked. Out of ninety B or C students, eighty-three eventually got an A and seven got a B.
>
> But that is not the way it is in other classrooms. If you get a bad grade on a paper, the students who got an A won't associate with you. If they associate with you, the teacher might think that they are hanging out with stupid people.

This method sounds quite logical. The A student keeps on learning and has to study because she in turn becomes the advocate for her partner, as in a mentor-mentee relationship. Meanwhile, she learns a lot about teamwork. Each member has strengths and weaknesses.

Needless to say, Gasparis Vonfrolio got a lot of flack from her colleagues. Why? She did things differently. Her method was not the "normal" way of teaching:

> I didn't have the students do care plans, because all they needed to do was copy them from their books and have them typed. That's called being a secretary. I would not allow any note taking in my

classes. Instead, I hired a court stenographer. What she did was record my lecture and transcribe it that night. Then I would have copies passed out to the students. My objective was to create a network of support among my students, so that when they were out working in the nursing profession, they would expand their own networks.

Gasparis Vonfrolio taught at the college for eight years. She began her teaching in the associate's program and then was moved up to the baccalaureate program. I asked if she was able to measure the results of her methods. She said that when she began, students' scores on the state boards were low. When she implemented her teaching techniques, the pass rate increased from 73 percent to 92 percent.

She Bugs You

All of us, at some time in our careers, have worked with people who drove us nuts. Why? You name it. But when it comes to working and developing teams, you don't have to like the people you work with. And liking you is not in their job description, either. People's only responsibility is to complete the tasks and functions they were hired for.

If you work with someone who bugs you, ask yourself why. Make a list. Annoying habits and irritating mannerisms can be ignored. Quality of work cannot. If the issues have to do with work, you may have to confront her.

Then identify and list her strengths. Why do you think she was hired. What are her skills? Separate the personal issues from the professional ones.

Finally, ask yourself, "What's in it for me to work with her? What's in it for her to work with me?" Don't think about whether you want to be friends. Consider her talents instead. If her work involves your work, wouldn't you like to see her accomplish what she needs to do, before it all comes crashing into your arena? If her mannerisms, habits, or traits have no impact on whether she gets her job done, then move on.

The Grumpies at Work

In every workplace there are morning people and night people. If you are a morning person and a few of your co-workers are night people and act like sourpusses when they come in each day, you have a problem. If you work with someone who seems to have a huge chip on her shoulders, then her style, her attitude, and her nonstop criticism may surround you like a giant thundercloud.

A bad attitude is not like a bad hair day. It doesn't change with something as simple as a shampoo and set. Something has to be done. If you are the team leader, part of your responsibility is to keep the group's productivity at a certain level. If someone's actions are dragging it down, it's up to you to stop the behavior before other team members start turning on each other, as well as on her—and, believe it or not, on you.

Get out your note pad. Start to write examples down, and cite lots of them. You will need to confront her privately. Don't expect a one-time mention to change her. You will probably have to repeat your examples at a later confrontation. If she denies her behavior, don't be surprised. She has been doing it for a long time. It's part of her.

The bottom line is that action is needed. When a co-worker has a bad attitude, it can destroy a team.

Identifying Saboteurs

There is no question that team members can and do sabotage others. Here are ten questions you can ask yourself, to uncover a saboteur in your midst. A *yes* to any one of them demands that you go on the alert.

Is There a Saboteur in the Midst?

1. *Does anyone keep a tally sheet?* Everyone makes mistakes. Saboteurs usually keep count and make a big brouhaha out of a small incident.

2. *Does anyone encourage gossip?* Most saboteurs are messengers. They can hardly wait to pass along damaging information about anyone or anything.

3. *Does anyone feel her job is in jeopardy?* Anytime fear and anxiety surface, as during downsizing, people overreact.

4. *Does information pass you by?* A common strategy of the saboteur is to isolate others, withholding information or interrupting the information pipeline.

5. *Is anyone on your team a bit too helpful?* Until you really know how your group operates, an overhelpful player may not be what you think she is.

6. *Does anyone stand to profit by another's mistake?* Saboteurs relish others' errors. These may be factors in a setup, and the saboteurs will benefit through promotions or bonuses.

7. *Have new coalitions formed on your team?* Saboteurs continually realign their "friendships."

8. *Does anyone bypass your authority and go over your head?* Saboteurs will do almost anything to look good, including sidestepping a leader's authority or ignoring other team members' contributions.

9. *Does anyone routinely deny involvement in certain activities yet know all the details?* Saboteurs can be chameleons, initially claiming no knowledge of an incident and yet passing details and information on to others.

10. *Does anyone encourage others to take on tasks that appear impossible?* Saboteurs take great pleasure in other people's mistakes and failures.

After identifying possible or probable saboteurs, your next step is to deal with them. When you confront, you need facts to back up your accusations. Most saboteurs will do just about anything to avoid exposure. They rarely commit anything to paper, and so you will need to have your facts together.

When a saboteur's motivation is redirected, you may be able to get your team back on track. Saboteurs don't like to be left out in the cold for long. They may actually attempt to make amends and rejoin "your" team.

Finally, the old saying "If you give her enough rope, she will hang herself" may apply. Once you identify your saboteur, you must side-step her games. Being a saboteur takes a lot of time and commitment. Over time, the saboteur will look and be less productive. The longer her game goes on, the less she produces, and the more likely she is to be exposed to others.

Teams are not created overnight. Most take months or even years to pull together. As the entire healthcare system enters a phase of change, the development of cohesive teams becomes a critical factor in defining and redefining an organization's vision and mission. Hospitals, associations, institutions, and businesses all have stated missions. Any organization that evolves from being individual-centered (I know what to do) to being leader-centered (You tell me what to do) and to being purpose-centered (We have a joint mission) will survive and grow with change.

11

Cultivate Healthy Female Relationships

A crucial step toward empowerment in the workplace is to develop and cultivate healthy relationships with other women. Women have entered the work force in unprecedented numbers. Contrary to popular belief and to some articles in the media, few women are really leaving. The Small Business Administration estimates that there are in excess of five million women-owned businesses today. This means that, no matter where you work, the odds are you will be working with other women.

In healthcare, as we have seen, the great majority of employees are women, and with over one-third of our 1993 survey respondents stating a preference not to work with other women, there are going to be problems. When women work together, there appear to be two camps, the good one and the bad one. The women who are in the good camp are more likely to be open about their positions, supportive of other women, and caring. They are confident about their skills and assertive, and they advocate advancing other women. The other camp, the bad one, is viewed as the troublemaker. The women within it tend to be more distant and uninvolved with group activities, are perceived to be at the heart of most rumors, and view other women not as their competitors but as their rivals. They are the type that is more likely to take credit for someone else's work, as well as not to acknowledge or applaud the work of others.

There are three primary relationships in which women work with other women. The first one is on the colleague–co-worker level, such as in nursing, drug sales, or marketing. The second will be between someone who is in management and a worker or employee. The third involves an indirect employer or employee connection (a woman doctor working with a staff nurse).

When women work with other women, confusing friendships with friendliness can and does create mayhem. Women too easily cross the line. There are work friendships that should remain within the work-related environment. Going out with other female nurses, co-workers, and doctors for a drink or playing in the summer softball or volleyball league continues the "work" flavoring. The crossover to family and more personal activities complicates the picture.

Female work friendships can be as complicated and, in some cases, as painful as workplace romances. Work friendships can create immense conflicts between work and personal life. This doesn't mean that all female relationships should be capped and not extended to your personal "other" life. It does mean that you need to be careful— that friendships are privileges and are built and earned over time. Few people meet and instantly fall in love. The great majority of positive, caring, and growing relationships have substantial investments of time in them.

In direct or indirect employee-employer or colleague–co-worker relationships, it's time to ask some serious questions. There are always the "right" or "politically correct" responses, but those are rarely your gut-level reactions to real-world situations. The Friendship-Savvy Quiz (Exhibit 11.1) asks ten questions, to be answered *yes* or *no* — with your gut reaction, not necessarily the one you know would be politically correct or expected in dealing with women in your workplace. Answering *yes* to any of the questions indicates that your personal expectations of others can be a damper on your own work, as well as on that of others. Women need to recognize that healthy relationships are a necessity—and that friendships, *real* friendships, are a luxury.

Exhibit 11.1.   Friendship-Savvy Quiz.

1. Would you feel uncomfortable if you needed to criticize her work?

2. Would you allow her extra time to complete tasks or projects?

3. Would you feel hurt or be angry if she took another position without telling you about it first?

4. Would you feel left out if she transferred to another department or moved to another city?

5. Would you feel excluded if she went to lunch with another co-worker and didn't invite you?

6. Would you feel overlooked or forgotten if she forgot your birthday?

7. Would you feel bad or uncomfortable if she criticized your work?

8. Would you feel betrayed if she told another a personal story or revealed anything that you considered intimate?

9. Would you feel uncomfortable competing for a position or promotion with her?

10. Would you cover for her if you knew she was having personal problems?

How Do Women Build Positive Relationships?

In the case histories that follow, you will see how women working together are learning to speak up, compete, confront, and collaborate—actions that are the building blocks of healthy relationships.

Women Doctors

As a supervisor, Cam sees a difference in how male and female doctors work with their colleagues, as well as with their patients. Cam's sentiments are echoed by others; there is far more collaboration among women doctors:

> Overall, I believe women doctors collaborate with their patients and the nurses. There are, of course, always exceptions. One female doctor has learned what she needs to do to get what she needs or wants. We don't have a lot of female doctors, but the ones we have appear to be kinder to their patients. They talk and listen to them. I don't believe that there is the arrogance among female doctors that male doctors routinely display.

As an administrative secretary in a hospital, Kimberly witnessed changes as soon as women doctors began to join the staff. Before that, she didn't see a lot of doctor-patient interaction. The women have changed it:

> The female doctors tend to refer their patients for additional information, have more follow-up, and tend to be more open about the whole concept of providing healthcare information to their patients. They also want to teach them to be more aware and to be a part of making decisions in their own care. In the past, the male doctors just have not done that.

In the intensive-care unit, Marilyn has seen dramatic changes in the interaction of women doctors and nurses:

Women doctors are great. First of all, they are much more down to earth, less godlike, and they work very hard. They are bright and have a good relationship with the nursing staff. In our unit, they collaborate on the different issues involving patients. The male doctors are still handing down edicts.

Sally, a nursing assistant, agrees with Marilyn. She feels that the women doctors get along better with patients and the nursing staff:

It seems like more of a collaborative effort, as far as working with the nurses is concerned. The women doctors really talk a problem over to find a solution.

A nurse manager, Mary Ellen, now goes to a woman doctor herself:

I now go to a woman physician, and my children go to a women pediatricians. I've found them to be fine doctors. All of us have been treated well. It's rare that I hear of any incident in the hospital where women physicians create problems for the nurses. The male doctors haven't changed much. In my opinion, they are among the most underdeveloped groups, socially, in the work force.

When I asked Mary Ellen about what kinds of socialization problems the male doctors had, her responses echoed those of other nurses. The male doctors threw temper tantrums, blamed nurses, and wrote derogatory comments to them on order sheets. One even wrote a letter to the nursing vice president, complaining about a nurse who consulted with him about a patient and then reported their joint observations and conclusions in the progress notes on the patient's chart. The doctor was incensed that she had done so without his permission.

Dorothy sums up her own reaction to women doctors: it's just easier. As a nursing supervisor, she has had the opportunity to work with them and evaluate the doctor-nurse working relationship:

> There is a much more relaxed relationship—more of a camaraderie with the women, versus working with the male physicians. With a man, you have to approach him correctly and make it look like "it's" his idea, whatever it is, even though you planted it in the first place. With the women doctors, it's totally different. You just state the way you think it ought to be, and they just say yes or no. We don't have the confrontations and conflicts that we routinely have with the male doctors.

It has been several years since Ursula worked in a clinical situation. Today, she is a nursing quality-assurance manager, and she has little opportunity to interact with physicians on a day-to-day basis, but she reports that she has noticed a difference since there have been more women doctors working in the hospital:

> Today I see the women doctors and the nurses being friendlier to one another. They call each other by their first names, which the male doctors do not encourage. Male doctors still want to be waited on. From what I see, there haven't been a lot of changes with the male doctor–nurse relationship.

Some of the women doctors who were interviewed indicated that not everything was perfect in their working relationships with nurses. As an RN for several years and now an emergency-room doctor, Kim sees a lot of friction between female physicians and nurses:

> Most recently, I've seen envy of some of the nurses toward the female healthcare workers. I believe it comes from their nonunderstanding of why another female in the hospital has more power than they do.

Kim also believes that there is still a problem with the general public's acceptance of women as physicians rather than nurses:

> They expect to see women as nurses or lab technicians, but not
> doctors. It's not that they dislike it. Rather, they just don't
> recognize that we are there.

Kim has experienced some variations in different parts of the country:

> In the South, patients expect a woman doctor to act like a
> nurse — to be softer and caring, not to give orders or tell them
> what they have to do. Where I practice, a great many patients
> never go outside a twenty-square-mile radius their entire life. The
> only contact they have with the outside world is television. And
> many of these people firmly believe that you don't take orders
> from women.

Margaret also has her practice in a southern state. When I asked her whether there are differences between male and female physicians and their working relationships with nurses, she responded that there are:

> Overall, I don't see the nurses here cooperating as well with the
> women doctors as they do with the men. I believe that a lot of the
> nurses view themselves as women doctors' rivals, not as our
> helpers or assistants. They are far more inclined to help the men.

Rita, a general surgeon, believes that women physicians spend more time with their patients across the board. She also feels that they show more empathy and compassion for their patients and the circumstances they are in. Communication is essential in the healing process, and Rita admits that some women physicians do not communicate as well as others. This should not be surprising. There are certainly some male doctors who do a fine job of communicating with their patients, their staff, and other medical professionals:

> Generally, women physicians spend far more time with their patients. The women that I personally know would all say that they are more compassionate than their male colleagues. Now, I also know women physicians who are abrupt and can be just as hard to deal with as some of my male counterparts. I think that's because of their training.

As an administrator, Gloria hears a lot of the hospital scuttlebutt. She is interested in the changes that the female physicians have brought to her workplace. She has noticed there is a difference in the newer physicians and how they interact with the staff:

> The older female physicians had to fight to get through school. I've noticed that their attitude with the staff is more likely to be "I'm the doctor, and you're the nurse." The younger and newer physicians are a little bit more relaxed. They view their work with the nursing staff as using a more team-oriented approach. I feel the younger generation of doctors will change our workplace for the better.

Donna, a nursing supervisor, talked about one of her hospital's physicians, who used to be an RN:

> There had been reports that she was more demanding of the nurses. Many had labeled her a bitch. The reality is that she is a little bit more demanding of them because she knows what the work expectations are. After all, she has been in their shoes. Since she's only been out of medical school for a few years, she watches herself, because she doesn't want to screw up. The bottom line is that she wants things done correctly.

Donna added that she doesn't see women speaking out against men when they screw up; they are more likely to speak up when another woman does. She also noticed some discrepancies in which doctors are called in an emergency:

> Many times, the male doctors don't want to work off-hours. They would rather sit home and watch the football game. The nurses would then call the female doctors. They really got blasted with emergency situations.
>
> I've also noted that the women doctors are not as quick to jump on the nurses or reprimand them for not coming to their rescue and helping them out as they would the male doctors. Patientwise, women patients love the female physicians. They feel that they understand what they need.

Donna concurs with other women who were interviewed in her observation that women doctors listen:

> I find it very refreshing to have female physicians in our practice. They bring a whole different twist to how we interact with our patients. These ladies don't make any bones about a situation. If they don't think something is right, they are more inclined to say, "Cut the bullcrap." They talk to the nurses as human beings, and they understand some of the frustrations we experience with patients as people, not just as bodies with an illness. The women will call a jerk a jerk.

Robyn has been in general practice for many years. Several of her patients are nurses, and she thinks that she gets along well with nurses, for the most part:

> I believe a lot of older women prefer working for a man. Part of it is age. I know for me it's much easier to work with people my age or younger than to work with people who are older.

When I worked for a male physician as an employee doctor, the nurse and staff, all women, would work for him but not for me. I remember asking one of the nurses to do something for me. She just left the room. I believe it's a generational thing. Older women prefer working for a man, and his age doesn't matter. They feel much more comfortable.

They used to get really ticked off when my patients called me by my first name. It's never been a big deal to me to be called Doctor, but to them it was very important. The woman who is now my partner is nine years older than I am. She believes that patients should call her Doctor.

Building Respect

The newest generation of female doctors is far more positive about nurses than the women doctors who completed their residencies more than ten years ago. Peggy is representative of many of the women doctors we interviewed. She recalls being a resident and doing a surgical rotation with another woman in a community hospital. Some nights were hard, but at times she was actually able to get five to six straight hours of sleep. Shannon, her fellow resident, didn't:

> Shannon is a wonderful person. But she knows how to annoy nurses better than anyone I know. She started on the rotation a few weeks after I did, and she came to me after a few days. She said she was getting stupid phone calls every half-hour, and it was a pain in the ass. I had to bite my tongue, because she didn't see that she was pissing off the nurses, and they were getting back at her. The first rule I learned is keep the nurses on your side. They are the ones who really have the power around here. Once you piss them off, you're in trouble.

Doctors like Peggy view nurses as an intricate part of the team. The best way to work with nurses is to respect them as individuals and for the talent they bring. Through the years, Peggy has observed male interns, residents, and specialists handing down orders. Their style is more dictatorial. Unfortunately, she says, some of the women doctors behave the same way the men do:

> I have a great deal of respect for nurses. At times, though, I believe the women doctors and nurses get into a type of competition. I've also been on the receiving end, when nurses sometimes had a problem accepting orders from me. It's only from the female nurses that I have had problems, when I've given orders and they haven't wanted to take them. When I observed their interactions with the male interns and residents, I didn't see the problems that I had.

What Peggy understands is that there are times when there will be competition between women in the workplace. Peggy feels that when the competitive spirit rears its head, the best way to resolve the problem is to defuse it. Her way is to actively work with the nurses and reinforce the fact that they are on her team:

> When I did my first internship, it was in a neonatal nursery. I'd never even been in a neonatal nursery before, much less worked in one. There were nurses who had worked there for twelve years. The reality was they could run that nursery just fine without me. I would have been an idiot to think that I always knew what was best. Anytime that orders needed to be written, I got into the habit of sitting down with whoever the nurse was and saying, "What do you think?" Doctors who don't think they can learn from nurses are crazy. I think most nurses are dynamite. I can't tell how many times I've had my tail saved by good nurses over the years.

Peggy finds it strange that so many doctors, particularly men, routinely exclude nurses from patient-care dialogues:

Let's say I have a patient with diabetes. I'm so focused on her diabetes that I welcome the nurses' input. One nurse may say that this patient could really do well with this instead of that. Another may think of comfort measures that I'm overlooking. Nurses also really know what to look for, and they catch which drugs interact with one another and which don't. I see having great interaction with nurses as part of good basic patient care.

Peggy was also one of the few respondents to the survey who acknowledged having been accused of unethical behavior. The incident occurred when she and her partner were doing routine physical exams on children in a psychiatric hospital:

> As a rule, we would have the nurse bring the child down to the examining room. Usually, she did not stay with us.
>
> As part of the routine, and because of the background of many of these kids, I would do a genital exam. I'd always tell the child beforehand and say the reason was to look for any medical problems. If the child said no, I would never push it.
>
> There was one little boy who was five or six years old, who told the nurse later that I had fondled him. The director of nursing contacted me and said, "I know you didn't abuse this child, and I'm not going to let this go any farther. I did want you to know that he was using words about sexual abuse that he shouldn't know at this age."
>
> The nurses reaffirmed their support for me. In the future, they would always make sure that there was someone in the room with us, so everyone would be protected. It was presented in a very supportive and caring way. I felt that they were there for me.
>
> I have to admit that it really threw me, and I was nervous during the next few exams. It's very scary, because many of these kids are neurologically messed up. Or the kids are actually okay,

but their families are screwed up. There are times I felt like I was treating the wrong patient.

Peggy's rules for dealing and working with nurses are designed to build positive relationships. But the building is not something that is done overnight. It takes time, even years. But by treating people with respect, honoring their diversity, not purposely getting others angry, and living and working with integrity, we can make our workplaces far more pleasant.

When it comes to women working with women, we definitely can be more open, honest, and supportive with each other. At the same time, we can compete and be assertive without viewing all other women as rivals. When women are confident about who we are and what we are, we do not have a problem with other women stretching, reaching, and growing. We welcome it. It will be women, not men, who redefine what it means for women to work with women.

12

Banish Geisha Nursing (and Other Female-Dominated Professions)

If a geisha is a girl or woman trained as an entertainer to serve as a hired companion to men, then a geisha nurse is one who flirts with or displays physical or verbal affection or submissiveness toward a male, usually a doctor. In August 1992, I had the opportunity to speak and work with a group composed of women physicians. They covered every facet of medicine and came from almost every state. In a workshop focusing on confidence and crises, the term *geisha* nursing surfaced. Many of the participants in the group were familiar with the term. They rolled their eyes and shook their heads as several women began to discuss the topic. It was one that I was not familiar with, but the phrase alone intrigued me.

As I probed further, first by listening and then by joining in the talk, I found that geisha nursing was indeed a factor. Elizabeth, one of the women physicians we interviewed, said she also had a geisha receptionist:

> She had discovered that her key way of getting along with men was to please them and be a flirt. I also find that women who display this tendency are the same ones I have the most conflict with.

Elizabeth has discovered that when people have trouble with authority or with accepting others' authority over them, they usually act from a submissive posture. The old rules of society say that it's all right to act submissively toward a man, but not toward a woman. If a man flirts with a woman who is submissive, it's acceptable. Women usually don't flirt with other women. When a woman attempts to assert authority over another woman, if there is going to be a negative reaction, it will mainly be unassertive or indirect.

In the emergency room, Natalie sees the same thing. In fact, she has reached the point where she enjoys it when a temporary male nurse is assigned:

> When we have a guy come on as a temp, he doesn't get caught up in the games—the male-female games. I find it refreshing.

Rosanne, chief of urgent care at a large health maintenance organization, had plenty to say. She had been an RN before going to medical school and had been a nurse manager. She said that if policies had been set by a male manager, no one would have questioned them. But because she was female, she felt, she was hassled. In her position, she was legally (and, in her opinion, morally) obligated to follow up on any reports of sexual harassment. When she did her job, she found that there were sometimes repercussions. Once, she told administrators that it was very difficult for her to work there as a woman. They suggested that she create a presentation that would increase the hospital's awareness.

Rosanne decided to interview all the women physicians in the facility, incorporating their concerns and feedback for the various departmental chiefs, all men. She titled her presentation "Geisha Nursing," primarily to get the administration's attention. She did:

> One of the key factors that the women physicians had identified involved working with nurses who preferred the 1950s style of

flirtatious interaction. The women nurses reacted violently to the title and content of my presentation, but I found geisha nursing so prevalent that I didn't know any other way to deal with it except to bring it out in the open.

In my department, I had over fifty physicians who rotated in and out on any given day. Of these, the great majority were men. There were forty on the nursing staff. When I was working with both groups, trying to change some schedules, I uncovered a series of complaints from women providers who were not getting nursing support, especially from the flirtatious ones.

The emergency-room doctors often worked as lone cowboys in their departments. They had a bevy of nurses whom they pretty much ordered around and had follow them around. The doctors who cracked chests needed a great deal of one-to-one support, and they got it. Then there were doctors who worked in the clinic. They didn't get the support the others did. Anyone related with emergency and surgery was showered with support staff, who trailed after their every move.

The way the other doctors coped with the groups who got the support was to cultivate special and flirtatious relationships with the nurses, so that they would get increased attention and aid. When I brought this up at a routine departmental meeting, I mentioned that we had to divide up time equally or allocate time on the basis of the acuity of patients' problems. We couldn't allocate time according to personal preferences.

The nursing staff said, "We are just nice to the people who are nice to us." They viewed flirtation as being nice. I responded that we couldn't do that—this was a professional setting, and flirting was both demeaning and inappropriate.

I went on to say that I would deal with the doctors and be an advocate for any nurse who needed help handling a doctor who displayed inappropriate behavior toward her. I wanted them to let me know, so that they would not have to succumb to the demands of powerful physicians. They were horrified. They rebelled and complained that I was souring the work environment.

What Rosanne told us is that the 1950s are alive and well. In the hospital environment, there is almost a caste system. One of the ways to move up and out of one's caste is to develop some type of bond with someone more powerful. In the hospital, doctors are powerful, and a nurse in a nurse-doctor liaison gets more status. Rosanne had assumed that the nurses would not want the doctors to flirt with them or take advantage of the intensity of the work environment. She assumed wrong. The geisha nurses liked it.

Rosanne also noticed that male doctors were allowed to display certain types of behavior that most people would call eccentric. A woman doctor behaving in the same way might find her job on the line:

> Many of the male doctors are prima donnas. There were times when they would scream, yell, and throw things and then turn around and flirt with the nurses. Their temper tantrums would be seen as eccentric. Eccentricities were forgivable because doctors are such valued workers.
>
> I have also observed doctors' special relationships with nurses, to the point where the doctors would get backrubs—huge, large men sitting in the nurses' laps, grinding their butts into them at the nursing stations. In this day and age, that's pretty far over the edge.

When that type of blatant behavior is observable, someone is bound to complain, as Rosanne and other women doctors did:

> Every year, the doctors had a departmental Christmas party. They would go off to a fine restaurant. There would be alcohol, food,

dancing—all off site. It looked like a standard party. The problem surfaced when the women doctors started attending.

These parties were like something out of a 1950s Jack Lemmon movie. Everyone was three sheets to the wind, and bosoms were everywhere. There was lewd dancing, and no spouses were allowed, just the women nurses, male doctors, and the few women doctors.

The women doctors spoke up. The first year they complained, no one did anything. No one seemed to notice. The grapevine said the women doctors were puritanical.

The next year, the women doctors boycotted the party because they felt it was so offensive. Nobody noticed that they weren't there. In fact, feedback came back that it was the best party yet.

The third year, the women doctors suggested bringing spouses. They thought it would eliminate the outrageous behavior. This time, the nurses went over the edge: they didn't want spouses. The male doctors said that it would spoil everything, because this was the nurses' chance to fantasize and pretend that they were doctors' wives.

When that happened, I threatened to quit. The chief of our department was forced to resign. It's doubtful that anything like that will recur in our department. Unfortunately, it's moved on to another, more macho section—the orthopedic service.

The orthopedic service is heavily populated with patients who are college athletes, and there is big money for doctors. If there is going to be behind-the-scenes (or even in-the-scenes) action between male doctors and geisha nurses, this service will have more than its share, according to Rosanne.

There are many former basketball stars and college jocks in the orthopedic department. It's like the men's locker room. You see all these young tall guys who are into sports. The women flock to the department because they like working with them. What's interesting is to see how the nurses dress: skin-tight white jeans and things like that.

Orthopods make a lot of money, and they have more expendable income for their Christmas parties. They were actually putting alcohol in the water cooler during the holidays. For their party last year, they rented a huge limo with full bar service. Several other limos brought the women employees to an extravagant restaurant, where there was plenty of wine—definitely not a work setting.

The other departments don't do this. They may have a dinner and give the nurses gift certificates. Very little booze will be made available.

Rosanne says that a lot of the nurses view her as a "mini-Hitler," a woman who's making their workplace a cold place to be in, and not as much fun as it used to be. Rosanne recently hired another physician to share her duties. At times she feels overwhelmed and realizes that if she had been in another setting, her responsibilities would have entitled her long ago to an assistant, or at least a co-chief. The administration finally agreed to hire another physician when Rosanne threatened to quit.

Word went out that a man had been hired, and many saw him as the man on a white horse—someone who would come in and make things nice again, the way things used to be. Rosanne's agreement with him is that she will play "bad cop" and he will play "good cop." Their objective is to support each other:

It's difficult. The nurses want the women to be mother-managers. They want mothers. They want to be overly personal. From men, they want sexual overtones. What's interesting to see is that many of the nurses act in a coquettish manner, and my co-chief doesn't respond to them, or at least not the way they expect. There are even rumors that I turned him into a bad person.

When women play games, we play them well. We have played them for centuries. It's not something that will be changed overnight, but it can be changed. Game playing that involves coquettish behavior is learned, not genetic.

As more and more women physicians enter the workplace, they will bring more of a no-nonsense approach. Verbal and physical harassment are being reported, and there is growing awareness that many women do not receive pay or promotions equal to those their male counterparts enjoy. More women are also entering surgery, including the macho field of orthopedics.

When nurses realize that their paychecks come from the combined revenues created by all doctors, not just a few men, geisha nursing should start to disappear. Until then, it will be a negative factor in the workplace. Recognizing it, and confronting behavior that is inappropriate and that undermines all work relationships, is one way to begin ushering it out.

13

Abolish Sexual Harassment

Sexual harassment was a taboo topic in the United States until Clarence Thomas was nominated for the Supreme Court in 1991, and Anita Hill brought it to everyone's attention. But the problem is not new. It dates back thousands of years. And sexual harassment is increasing. In 1990, 64 percent of all women in the military reported harassment, 75 percent in the Navy alone. On college campuses, 40 to 70 percent of female students experience harassment from male students. Elementary and high schools also report high levels of sexual harassment. It's no wonder that the workplace is a boiling pot of unwelcomed attention.

Nine out of ten victims of sexual harassment are women. In Susan Webb's excellent book, *Step Forward: Sexual Harassment in the Workplace,* she writes that the most common behavioral definition of sexual harassment is "Deliberate and/or repeated sexual or sex-based behavior that is not welcome, not asked for and not returned."[1] She goes on to say that this definition has three major elements and two qualifiers.

The first element is that the behavior in question has to be sexual in nature or sex-based. In other words, it's behavior with some sort of sexual connotation, or behavior that occurs because of the victim's being specifically a male or a female. The range of behavior with sexual connotations is very wide. The offender may not be interested in actually having sex. The spectrum encompasses the minor or least severe infractions (joking, innuendoes, flirting, asking someone for a date) and the more serious manifestations (forced fondling, attempted or actual rape, sexual assault).

The second element is that the behavior has to be deliberate and/or repeated. Some forms of sexual behavior are so graphic and offensive that the first time they occur they are considered deliberate, inappropriate, or even illegal. Forced fondling, attempted rape, and serious sexual slurs are examples. Other forms of behavior must be repeated over and over before they become harassment. Telling jokes may not offend one person, but another may find the jokes insulting or degrading. And the jokes may not be annoying initially. In a few days, weeks, or months, however, they cease to be funny or amusing to the person who is subjected to them. Legally, the behavior may not be sexual harassment, but it still takes a toll on its target.

The third element is that the behavior is not welcomed, asked for, or reciprocated. Behavior that two people mutually engage in for their own enjoyment is simply that—mutual. As long as it doesn't interfere with their work or create an objectionable environment in the workplace, it is usually permissible. Many view the responsibility for setting limits as the victim's: "It can't be sexual harassment unless she or he says it is." Maybe.

The first qualifier can be stated as follows: the more severe the behavior is, the fewer times it has to be repeated before reasonable people define it as harassment; the less severe it is, the more times it has to be repeated. The severity of the behavior must be considered in conjunction with the number of repetitions.

The second qualifier is as follows: the less severe the behavior is, the more responsibility the target has to speak up (because some people do like this kind of behavior); the more severe it is, the less responsibility the target has to speak up (the initiator of the behavior should be sensitive enough in the first place to know that it is inappropriate). Light harassment tends to get worse and becomes severe when it's not addressed and stopped early on.

Sexual harassment may be verbal, nonverbal, or physical. The most common verbal forms are jokes, insults, comments, and remarks. Nonverbal harassment can be just as intimidating. Use of certain kinds of gestures, looks (leering, ogling), cartoons, or photographs are common in this type of harassment. Physical harassment, which includes touching, pinching, rubbing, or "accidentally" brushing against someone's breasts or buttocks, is more severe and may involve criminal charges.

Sexual harassment is about power. The harasser believes or knows, consciously or unconsciously, that he (or she) has more power than the target. The person harassed also believes that the harasser has greater power. If the harasser did not believe he had more power, there would be minimal or no harassment. If the target did not believe it, she could turn to the harasser and demand that he stop.

Victims of harassment give two primary reasons why they file lawsuits or make formal complaints outside their organizations, rather than solving the problem at work: they *feel* powerless ("I didn't think anyone would take me seriously"), or they *are* powerless ("I couldn't get it stopped any other way.[2]

Sexual harassment can be broken into five types, each one more severe than the last:

1. General harassment (includes generalized sexist remarks and behavior)
2. Seductive behavior (inappropriate and offensive but essentially sanction-free behavior)

3. Sexual bribery (solicitation of sexual activity or other sex-linked behavior, with promise of rewards)

4. Sexual coercion (pressure for sexual activity by means of threats)

5. Sexual imposition or assault (inflicted sexual activity, such as touching, fondling, grabbing, assault, rape, or attempted rape)

Harassment in Medicine

In February 1993, a published survey of 133 young doctors revealed that three-quarters of the women and one-fifth of the men believed that they had been sexually harassed during their medical training. Most of the incidents involved offensive comments. Off-color jokes, remarks about people's anatomy, or persistent and unwelcome flirtation were the incidents most often cited.[3] The women reported that nearly all the unwanted attention had come from male doctors. The men said that they had most often been harassed by nurses (half of them males). One female resident said that she had been asked out on dates by two different doctors who were supposed to write letters of recommendation or evaluations for her. Another woman said that a senior resident had frequently rubbed his groin against her during operations. Women also reported continually being targets of leering, and they said that male doctors stood too close to them and gave them unwanted kisses and pats.

In one case of sexual bribery, a woman doctor said that she had been offered good grades and other advantages in exchange for sex. A few of the women said that they had reported the harassment to someone in authority, and that the incidents had been resolved. Three-quarters of the respondents had not reported the incidents, because they doubted they would get any help. The majority of the women said that the episodes had created an intimidating environment and interfered with their ability to work.

The Crotch Approach

Laura Gasparis Vonfrolio believes that if nurses will speak up and speak out, sexual harassment that involves leering, sexual innuendoes, and unwanted remarks can be halted. She admits that some of her tactics are outrageous, but she's found that they work:

> In one of the ICUs, there is a doctor who responds when you ask him to write an order, "If you jiggle your boobs, I'll write it." I cannot believe that nurses tolerate and allow this sort of interaction to go on. In our unit, several of us got together to discuss what we could do to prevent him from talking to us this way. I suggested that when he comes in, we should just stare at his crotch.
>
> The next time he came into our unit, everyone looked at his crotch. Nowadays, this man is in and out of our unit so fast he doesn't have time to talk to anybody.
>
> Initially, everyone was afraid to do it. When I asked why, no one really came up with a valid reason. I said, "Do you think he's going to go to the hospital administration and say, 'All the nurses are staring at my crotch'?" He would never do that. It's the first time in a long time the nurses from our unit have stuck together.

Gasparis Vonfrolio's recommendation may seem unorthodox, but when you are in an environment that caters to those in power—doctor's, especially male doctors—complaints to administrators usually are of no avail.

Women Can Be Harassers, Too

When Gloria experienced sexual harassment, she was one of a group of clinical nurse managers. Over a period of time, she learned that she was the only heterosexual woman in the group. She also found that she was frequently written up as a manager, was given special directives that others did not have to follow, had pay raises withheld, and was even put on probation. It was the first time in the history of her organization that a manager had been put on probation. Then one of the vice presidents stepped in and said, "Something is wrong. This doesn't fit." Gloria describes the situation as follows:

> Sexual preference has little to do with anything, unless it affects other people and doesn't let them do their job or move ahead in an organization. That's what I felt it was doing. At this point, senior management has taken a close look and has brought in consultants to deal with it.

Eventually, a new vice president for nursing was brought in and dramatically turned the situation around, at least for Gloria. But until that time, her workplace was toxic for five years:

> I tried to keep doing my job. I didn't confront it. Usually, I have no problem confronting male-to-female sexuality. I know how to handle that. But in this situation I didn't know how, and my job was in jeopardy. If I had it to do all over again, I would have stood up a lot sooner.

Today, Gloria routinely exercises with two of the top administrators from her hospital. One of them revealed that what Gloria encountered had been the basis of a recruitment problem for several years. Finally, a staff member sent a letter, saying that if the problem wasn't taken care of, she would go to the press.

What Gloria reported is no different from what many other women feel in the workplace. Whether it's in healthcare, in a service organization, or in manufacturing, there is a sense of isolation and a feeling that "it's only happening to me, and if I do speak up, it won't matter, because the administration doesn't listen."

Keep Your Fingers to Yourself

Cam, a staff RN and relief nursing supervisor, remembers times when doctors literally backed her out of rooms with their fingers, pushing and poking at her with each step. That was thirty years ago, and she did not speak up. Things are different now:

Similar incidents have occurred recently. Today, I can speak up and make it clear that this kind of behavior is out of line.

Her response should also include the announcement that she will not tolerate this behavior any longer, and that if it doesn't stop, she will report it.

Girls Don't Like It

Claudia, an OB/GYN nurse, works in surgery. She says that the male doctors frequently make sexual remarks:

Recently, a chest tube was being put into a baby girl. One of the male doctors said, "Put it in a little farther. Girls like that." I heard that remark when I started working in the hospital, when I was eighteen years old. Today I'm fifty-one. And these are educated, respected surgeons!

These surgeons are often married and the fathers of girls. What is interesting to note is that these comments are usually made when there are other men around—fellow doctors, medical students, or others they are trying to impress.

Don't Stereotype the Victim

Data have been accumulated about victims and harassers. A profile of a "typical" victim can be drawn up, but most experts in the field of sexual harassment feel that there is danger in describing what a typical case looks like. Once identified, a victim's actions become stereotyped. Assumptions surface: victims have control; if they didn't behave or look certain ways, they wouldn't be harassed. One of the myths of sexual harassment is that the victim caused it, and too often the victim gets blamed. Nevertheless, some general statements can be made about victims of sexual harassment:

- Most victims are female. Approximately 90 percent of incidents are experienced and reported by women.

- Female victims are younger than the general female population. The women are usually in their twenties or thirties (specifically, twenty-four to thirty-four for more severe forms of harassment).

- Women who are married or widowed are less likely to be harassed than women who are divorced, separated, or never married.

- Women who are well educated are just as likely to be harassed as less educated women.

- Male victims of sexual harassment are much more likely than female victims to be subjected to same-sex harassment.

- Male victims are generally older than their female harassers.

Many women and men don't fit this pattern, however. Victims are found in all age groups, marital-status groups, job categories, pay ranges, and racial and ethnic groups. Victims of sexual harassment report feeling angry, upset, frightened, guilty, embarrassed, demeaned, intimidated, trapped, powerless, defeated, or violated, whether they are female or male. Headaches, backaches, and stomach problems are common stress-related results. The end result is loss of ambition, decreased job satisfaction, and impairment of performance. Everyone loses.

Snapshot of a Harasser

The risk of stereotyping also exists in describing a harasser, of course, but people who are guilty of sexual harassment look something like this:

- Usually, harassers are male, older than their victims, married, and considered unattractive by their victims.

- Most harassers are co-workers, if for no other reason than the fact that most employees are nonsupervisory. The most severe and frequently reported harassment is directed by supervisors at their subordinates.

- Harassers frequently bother more than one person, and incidents recur over an extended period of time. The higher the percentage of men in a work group, the greater the amount of harassment directed at women.

- Motives for sexual harassment by men fall into three categories: actual sexual desire; desire for more personal power (by harassing, the man feels more important or virile); and desire for social control (the man who does not want women in the workplace harasses them to get rid of them or to put them in "their" place).

- Female harassers are involved in an estimated 1 percent of cases, and their victims are almost always men; female-to-female harassment is rare.

- Female harassers are usually divorced or single and younger than their victims.

- The "average" man who propositions or harasses a woman is much like the "average man" in the work force. The "average" woman who makes advances is not at all typical of the "average" working woman. She is more likely to be a supervisor than a co-worker.

The Victim Trap

Denial is one of the most common forms of discounting by the victim. She tells herself, and others, "He really didn't mean it that way" or "I must be misinterpreting his intentions" or "Surely he's not really coming on to me" or "This can't be happening; I must be crazy."

As harassment continues, why doesn't the denial stop? It's because sexual harassment is humiliating. When the harasser is a supervisor or a co-worker one likes, the humiliation is compounded. Denial enables the victim to avoid dealing with a painful situation.

Victims may recognize that they are being harassed but decide to do nothing: "It's just part of working here. You've got to expect it. It comes with the territory." Rarely does the problem go away. It gets worse, and the victims end up irritable, touchy, and less effective in their work.

Another common trap is that victims blame themselves. They may even attempt to look less attractive: "If I look less sexy, he will leave me alone." In most cases, looks have very little to do with it, and the harassment continues. Sexual harassment is not the victim's fault.

Victims sometimes blame others who are not involved. In this situation, other women or men in the office are blamed for "causing" the harasser to harass. This happens when it is difficult or risky for a victim to confront her harasser directly. If she did, her job or safety could be threatened.

Avoidance is a tactic sometimes used as a coping mechanism. Certain people, jobs, and places are avoided. When a victim spends work time trying to cope with inappropriate or illegal behavior, her job performance is affected. But she may feel that avoidance is the only realistic alternative.

Nevertheless, the only way to stop sexual harassment is to bring it out in the open. Victims must recognize sexual harassment for what it is, understand that it is not their fault, and know they have a right to complain and get it stopped.

She Made Me Do It

Harassers attempt to invalidate or discount claims of sexual harassment. When confronted by the victim or by someone else trying to help stop the harassment, the harasser may say that the victim has no sense of humor and can't take a joke. The victim complains that the jokes or remarks are not funny; they are offensive, embarrassing, often degrading. The harasser says that the employee who feels victimized is not a good sport and "just can't take it." Testing and teasing may be part of the social initiation that goes on in the workplace, but when testing or teasing are about sex, they become degrading or offensive.

Some harassers try to deny their actions by reinterpreting their own intentions or motives and claiming that the victim misunderstood. Webb calls this the "I was just" game. When the offending employee is asked or told to stop a certain behavior, he or she says, "I was just being nice" or "I was just teasing" or "I was just complimenting her." If there actually has been a misunderstanding, the victim is made aware of it, and the inadvertent offender learns to be more careful in the future. Blaming the victim for the harassment is the most common form of discounting—saying the victim asked for it, started it, wanted it, or that the victim is a bitch or a troublemaker.

Harassers in the Workplace

There are three kinds of harassers or potential harassers: unaware, insensitive, and hard-core. Most of us, at one time or another, fall into the *unaware* category. Things are said and done that embarrass others or make them feel bad. When we are aware that our actions have caused embarrassment, we stop. In turn, we are embarrassed by the situation. This kind of behavior should be called inappropriate instead of harassing. Once awareness of unintentional behavior is reached, it can be stopped by the victim.

Insensitive harassers are a bigger problem. They know that their behavior is offensive to others, and they continue, even though they have been asked and told to stop. Only someone with more power (a supervisor or manager) or a policy statement, combined with discipline, will stop the behavior.

Hard-core harassers are usually angry and hostile. They continually degrade, intimidate, embarrass, and abuse their co-workers. Because of their unwillingness to change their behavior, these individuals are being terminated and replaced. Organizations can't afford to keep them.

Dealing with Complaints

Complaints that involve an employee and an alleged harasser can be handled or resolved by a supervisor or manager, working only with the two people involved. A more complex complaint, one that requires actual investigation, is usually handled by a human resources professional or an outside investigator. Both the employees involved, as well as others who are witnesses or victims of harassment, will be included.

A simple complaint consists of four elements: an interview with the complaining employee and the alleged harasser; an evaluation of the incident(s); a review of any records; and immediate and appropriate action. During the evaluation, the supervisor or manager must take all the circumstances into account. Action taken against an employee should be appropriate to the offense; the punishment must fit the crime. Any supervisor or manager who handles complaints should be familiar with the typical responses and behavioral patterns of victims and harassers.

Stepping-Stones for Employees

Stopping sexual harassment may sound easy, but it's not. When sexual harassment occurs and you are a victim of it, you must put a game plan into effect. By laying out your plan and writing down your thoughts, feelings, and expected outcomes, you begin the move toward resolution.

First, it is imperative to admit there is a problem. Denial doesn't work. If you are an avoider in dealing with conflict, your normal response will be to ignore it and hope it will go away. Rarely does sexual harassment disappear of its own accord.

Second, recognize sexual harassment for what it is. It's deliberate and/or repeated, unwanted, unwelcome sexual behavior directed at you. Is the behavior being directed at you because of your gender? Is it happening on purpose, or is it accidental? Is it repeated over and over? Does the harasser know that it is unwelcome? Have you said or indicated that you don't like it? Do you participate in or initiate the behavior?

Third, bear in mind that the problem doesn't go away unless it's addressed. It may be a question of inappropriate behavior (repeated jokes or innuendoes) or of hard-core harassment ("put out or get out").

Fourth, no matter what the behavior is, it costs everybody. You pay in stress and reduced productivity. It's harmful personally and professionally.

Fifth, your organization should have an interest in stopping the behavior. Sexual harassment costs money, whether in low productivity, increased absenteeism, or low morale.

Sixth, accept responsibility for taking part in solving the problem. This does not mean that you are to blame.

Seventh, privately and calmly, tell the person that you don't like his or her behavior.

Eighth, use an "I" statement: "*When* you call me 'honey' (touch me, tell me jokes), I *feel* very upset (embarrassed, offended) *because* I want to be taken seriously (want to be treated as an equal, want respect).

Ninth, use the broken-record technique. It acknowledges the behavior, and then you repeat your "I" statement. If the harasser responds that he didn't mean to hurt your feelings, or that you may be too sensitive, say something like "I understand you didn't mean to hurt my feelings. However, *when* you did ____, I felt ____ because ____."

Tenth, say what you do or don't want done: "Please call me by my name (don't touch me, don't tell me those jokes)." Be specific.

Try these ten steps once or twice. If they don't bring any results, then you are going to have to take more steps. The harasser is not responding or ceasing his behavior. You need help.

First, ask a co-worker for support and even aid in talking with the offender. Sometimes the harasser can hear a message more clearly from a friend or a buddy.

Second, go to a supervisor or a manager to get additional help if the behavior does not stop after the confrontation.

Third, don't assume that the behavior will stop or go away if you ignore it. Sexual harassment gets worse when it is ignored.

Fourth, avoid dealing with severe harassment alone. In a serious case, let someone in the company know about it immediately. Get help.

If these four additional steps don't work, or if the problem appears to be escalating or becoming more complex, then you need a more detailed plan. It's critical for you to maintain your balance and perspective by assessing all the elements of the problem.

First, examine it. What does the other person say or do? What do you say or do? When, where, and how often does it happen? Does it happen to others? On a scale of 1 to 10, how severe do you consider each event?

Second, write down the answers to these questions. Writing them down will help you clarify the issues and give yourself objectivity. Write a description, as factual as possible, of each event.

Third, take a look at the other person and record your thoughts. What's going on with him? Why is he treating you this way? Is it possible that the other person is unaware of the negative effects that the behavior has on you? Is the other person trying to be friendly, or could he be truly attracted to you? Is this person aware of the effects of his behavior but uncaring and insensitive to your feelings or to how you've asked to be treated? Is this person treating you this way deliberately and maliciously, after your repeated objections?

Fourth, look at yourself. Have you been participating in the problem? This doesn't mean to dump the blame on yourself. You know that's a common trap. Just make sure you have considered all the aspects. Does your self-image at work project how you want to be treated? Have you said *no* directly and specifically to the harasser, so that there is no misunderstanding of your nonverbal messages?

Fifth, using your analysis of the problem, list all the ideas you can think of that can help stop the behavior. Then group or organize your ideas into plans: A, B, and C. Some of the ideas may be included in more than one plan.

Sixth, make your plan specific with regard to time, place, and actions. Think through all the consequences. Keep in mind that you have two simultaneous goals at this point: to get the behavior stopped, and to maintain your effectiveness in your job.

Seventh, include other people in your plans. Don't try to be a hero and handle it alone, especially with harassers who seem to be insensitive or malicious. Call on friends, supervisors, or managers who can be of help.

Eighth, keep your plans flexible. The response of the harasser or the manager may change your plans or your timetable. Solving this problem involves other people and their time and effort, not just your own. Be reasonable.

Ninth, implement plan A, B, or C, as necessary. If you have gone through the preceding steps, you should be able to put your plan into action more calmly and competently and get the results you want.

Stepping-Stones for Supervisors

When sexual harassment surfaces in the workplace, a supervisor or manager cannot bury her head or ignore it. Many organizations that ignored or treated a situation with "benign neglect" have paid substantial sums of money to harassed employees.

There are four circumstances in which supervisors have to deal with sexual harassment: when a complaint is made to them, when they hear about behavior they think may be harassment, when they see or hear about behavior that they know is harassment, and when they see or hear about others engaging in behavior that they think may be offensive.[4]

When an employee complains about sexual harassment, listen and find out what action she wants taken. It could be just to talk, to get more information about her rights, or to handle it alone. Offer to talk to the offending employee privately or to meet with the two of them together, if the victim wants a supervisor's help in resolving the problem.

Document briefly for yourself the who, what, when, and where of your discussion with the complaining employee. Notify your supervisor and/or the personnel or equal employment opportunity office. Follow up by checking back with the employee. Repeat this step as necessary.

Encourage the harassed employee to say *no* to the offender, but do not require the employee to handle the situation. Treat the offender's behavior as you would any other serious misconduct, by following your organization's disciplinary procedures. Correct and stop the inappropriate behavior immediately. Most lawsuits are filed as a last resort—the victim could not get the behavior stopped.

As a supervisor, you should not assume the victim is at fault or asked for it, discount or make light of the situation, encourage the victim to outwit or embarrass the harasser, tell the harassed employee to ignore the complaint, or allow the behavior to continue.

Sexual harassment is illegal. Most victims grin and bear it, rarely speaking up or speaking out. To eliminate it, women and men—employers and employees—must treat it as intolerable and inappropriate in the workplace. Period.

14

Get a Mentor, Be a Mentor

Being a mentor involves an interactive relationship with a mentee. A good mentor nurtures the evolving mentee. A good mother nurtures her young, too, but there is a difference between mothering and mentoring; what most women don't need is another mother in the workplace. Mothers often overprotect in their attempt to eliminate or reduce the risks their children encounter. A mentor empowers a mentee to take on the responsibilities and the risks that are in her path.

In the June 1993 *Working Woman* article on women bosses, three out of four of the top female wage earners stated that they make a special effort to mentor other women. In addition, two out of three of the top earners, those making over $75,000 a year, say that they speak out for women whenever possible; only 44 percent of the women earning less than $25,000 a year felt that women have an obligation to help other women.[1] In other words, the consensus was that the more you personally earn, the more you should give back.

A Mentor Is Your Advocate

Good mentoring relationships are always reciprocal. The mentee, the woman who receives guidance from her benefactor or sponsor, responds with support for her mentor. She receives information and ideas from her mentor, and others whom she works for benefit as the ideas are implemented.

Mentors are teachers, sponsors, advisers, coaches, guides, and counselors. Sometimes they are friends. As teachers and advisers, they help chart career paths for their mentees. As guides, they walk those paths with their mentees. In a healthy mentoring relationship, the mentor has been through the school of hard knocks. As a counselor, she uses her experience to help the mentee avoid some of the potholes that surface in the workplace. As a sponsor, she expands networking capabilities within the professional ranks. As a coach, she supplies emotional support when pitfalls are encountered. Many view mentors as role models, but there is a distinct difference. A role model can be anyone; there does not have to be a direct relationship.

Types of Mentors

Three types of women serve as mentors. The *traditional mentor* is usually older and more established in her career and in the organization. The *next-step mentor* is usually just one career level ahead of you and is closer in age. The *co-mentor* would be considered your peer and is often the same age. She is more of a collaborator on your career path.

Each type offers advantages. The traditional mentor brings power through her seniority. She has been around for a substantial period of time and is unlikely to lose out because of a political reorganization. When you are in a next-step mentoring relationship, all goes well if your mentor is "politically correct" in safe territory; otherwise, your relationship with her can be a handicap. One of the advantages of the co-mentoring relationship is that each woman brings strengths to the relationship, and they can propel each other toward whatever goals have been defined.

A mentor likes what she does. Her enthusiasm and energy are contagious. She is also very secure in herself and self-confident. She doesn't feel threatened when her mentee begins to outgrow the relationship—a common occurrence. If a mentee is bright and ambitious, or if her personal or career goals and visions change, her relationship with her mentor will change, and the relationship will need reassessment.

Don't Send In the Clones

Mentors have expertise in specific areas, and that's what mentees are looking for. Ideally, a mentor should be nonjudgmental and accepting of you as an individual, but it's not necessary for you to be her clone. Women who are excellent mentors encourage their mentees to move through their own space, with their own style. When the mentor looks in the mirror and is comfortable with the image that looks back, she can demonstrate her professionalism and leadership simply by being who she is.

Who Should Be a Mentor?

Jeanne Watson Driscoll, a psychiatric clinical nurse specialist, has been a mentor many times. She identifies several factors that enable a mentor to be helpful, including belief in the mentee, a commitment to investing her own time and expertise in the mentee's development, and the ability to recognize what the potential mentee can do for her.[2]

Women who are Queen Bees, with the attitude that you need to make it on your own, are women to be avoided as mentors. Phantom Bees, women who believe that *no one* is as competent or qualified as they are, should also be deleted from your list of potential mentors. Women who are not team players should be avoided, too. They can't offer the give-and-take that this relationship requires. Ideally, it is a win-win relationship: a woman mentor will see her own leadership skills grow, and her own carer planning and credibility may be enhanced.

Reaching out and offering her expertise and guidance to another woman encourages her to reevaluate her own career—where she is going, and what she wants to be at the end of the road. A healthy mentor encourages the mentee's transition from being nurtured to being empowered. When a mentee stretches and begins to reach her goals, a mentor is pleased that she has been the cheerleader and advocate.

Phases of Mentoring

In the beginning phase, the rules, written and unwritten, are laid out. Boundaries are determined. What's all right and what is not should be spelled out.

A woman who is a mentor is extraordinarily busy. You may not be the only mentee she has. Respect her time. Find out the best time to call her, and set up appointments. If you ask her early in your relationship how best to work with her, you will show her that you respect and honor her commitment to you. You can then adjust your time and needs to match hers. The odds of a successful mentorship will be significantly enhanced.

The middle phase is training. This is the time when you get to know each other. Your mentor does not have to be your friend. She doesn't even have to like you personally in order to respect you and recognize your potential. In the training phase, she is investing in you. Her words of wisdom and guidance during this time will become your tools, which will take you to your next level in the organization.

The final phase is termination. You may have outgrown your mentor, and it's time for you to move on. Or perhaps your mentor's goals, aspirations, or position with the company has changed. It's highly probable that a friendship has grown between you. Although you will both go your separate ways, there is a bond. A friendship that grows from a healthy mentorship is a bonus.

The Toxic Mentor

As in any other kind of relationship, there can be problems. The relationship may become unbalanced: the mentee may become totally dependent on her mentor for approval or authority, or the mentor may become dependent on the mentee for attention, admiration, and support. A mentee may feel that she is being exploited by her mentor, or that her mentor is trying to control her and even sabotage her efforts. This kind of mentorship is not healthy. For example, several of the women interviewed for this book had seen a mentor take credit for their work. Others said that their mentors were open, supportive, and encouraging but were mysteriously unable to offer help or information at the moment when it was needed.

Toxic mentors can derail your career, and they come in several varieties. *Cloggers* leave you out of the loop. *Wreckers* initially take pride in what you do and what you have achieved, and then suddenly nothing you do is right, and no matter how wonderful you think it is, they will find the flaw. *Castoffs* have a bit of the Queen Bee in them. Their attitude is often "Sink or swim," and when they finally decide to help, it's usually too late. *Escape artists* talk a good line. They tell anyone and everyone that they are mentoring you and have high hopes for your advancement, but they are never around when you need them.

Toward Empowerment

Women need to recognize their potential to be mentors, and they must be willing to be mentors. Mentoring is one key to eliminating some pitfalls of the workplace.

When a woman agrees to serve as your mentor, she puts you on the road to empowerment. But empowerment isn't something that can be given to you. It is *learned* and *earned* along your path. At times, you will get extra doses. At other times, you will have setbacks and feel disempowered.

A man can mentor a woman but a woman is probably better. Women don't need to be mini men, even if they do need men's knowledge and experience. But when women mentor other women, they demonstrate that they care about women's future and participation in the work force.

If you are new in your workplace, keep your eyes and ears open. Find out who has skills, expertise, respect, and power in your present environment, as well as in the area you would like to progress to. Find a woman you would like to emulate. Seek her out, and let her know that you respect and admire her. (Everyone loves flattery, as long as it's not excessive.) Ask for a fifteen-minute appointment, or invite her for coffee (and don't forget—you pay).

Many people feel that a woman in a strong position should automatically reach down and make time for other women. The woman herself may also feel that way, but she has a constraint—time. Bear in mind that she is busy and has a lot of responsibilities. That's why she holds the position she does.

After you solicit her support and she agrees to act as your guide and advocate, remember that you need to support her and respect her time. Let her make the rules.

While you're reaching up, extend your hand down, and become a mentor to another woman. Mentoring does take time and commitment. If you offer your hand to another woman, or to several, you have taken on a responsibility that is not light. Define your rules, just as your mentor did.

Whether you are the mentor or the mentee (and many women

are both), the relationship will be career-focused. If a friendship develops over time, congratulations. That's your bonus. It's not a prerequisite or a required outcome.

When women take it upon themselves to act as mentors to other women, they ensure that women's views and voices will be actively and enthusiastically passed on to future generations—another step toward empowerment.

15

Embrace Change

According to futurist Faith Popcorn, we will change as much in the 1990s as we did in the fifty years from 1940 through 1990. In the five years from 2000 to 2005, the equivalent of another fifty years of change will be experienced. In other words, Popcorn says, any of us who have lived through the fifteen years from 1990 to 2005 will actually have lived through one hundred years of change.

Faced with change in the workplace, it is not uncommon for people to go through five stages: resistance, skepticism, adaptation, shifting, and cohesiveness. In the stage of *resistance*, people will do whatever they can to ward off change, when change is the only reality. *Skepticism* brings stress, but the stress is somewhat eased in the *adaptation* stage (best characterized by the adage "Try it—you might like it." The *shifting* stage is still uncomfortable, and sometimes the "good old days" seem good indeed. At the stage of *cohesiveness*, the change— whatever it is—has been accepted, often so comfortably that the past is hard to imagine.

People tend to take three positions on change, too: reactive, non-active, and proactive. People who are *reactive*, jump out of the way. They'd rather not get involved. Those who are *nonactive* stand still;

they are paralyzed. People who are *proactive* get involved. They ask questions and create their own future, rather than having someone else create it for them.

Walking on Eggshells

The women interviewed for this book say that change is everywhere in healthcare—change coupled with fear. For example, I spoke with Melissa twice. A follow-up call was made two months after her initial interview. I asked if there had been any changes since I had last talked with her at the hospital where she worked:

> In the last two months, we are all walking on eggshells. At every meeting we have, a recurrent theme— "We just don't know what's going to happen"—surfaces. People speculate how much we'll have to trim, and what's going to be affected by cutbacks. We are very fearful.

Many women felt that the projected healthcare reform would be extremely hard for and on women. As a rule, women in healthcare have less power, and so they most likely will have less input on any changes that do occur. Rita, one of the women surgeons, sees desperate behavior among doctors and administrators:

> Everyone feels very threatened and is panicking. People feel that they are losing control and are snapping at anyone who gets in their way. They are less patient with everybody and everything.

A great many of the women felt that their hospitals existed only for profit and had forgotten about taking care of people. Margaret, an internist, feels that hospitals have lost sight of their mission:

> They have become greedy. I can remember a time when they used to have nonprofit hospitals, whose mission was primarily to take care of people. Today, hospitals have lost their vision of what they

are supposed to be doing. I see them doing all this fancy marketing, and charging huge prices. I'm really not thrilled with the hospitals. They have caused a lot of their own problems.

Too Many Layers

The general consensus among those interviewed was that healthcare will have to move toward prevention and farther away from treating sickness. Many saw their units moving from inpatient to outpatient care. They felt that money should be focused on women and children, where prevention would be most effective. The consensus was also that too much money was being spent on high technology, and that financial and technology-related abuse was pervasive. Many felt that there were too many chiefs, and some thought their organizations were just too big.

Maureen has worked for thirty years. She holds bachelor's and master's degrees and began her work in radiation oncology. Today she is a senior nurse manager in a large nonprofit hospital. She believes her hospital is no different from any other in trying to reduce costs:

> We were recently asked to look at ways to cut back. The head of dietary said she could cut back on some cheap people, those who deliver the trays. What happens then is that the nurses are expected to deliver trays.
>
> I believe that people forget that hospitals are like a mobile in a baby's crib. If you remove one of those pieces, the rest of the mobile slants to one side. That's what I see happening in the hospitals. I believe the pieces that have to be removed are some of the layers that are higher up in the hospital.

Maureen would begin at the departmental level, from the department head on up. In her hospital, the president doesn't even maintain an on-site office:

When the president comes to our hospital, he needs someone to show him around. On-site officers are the chief executive officer and the chief operations officer, who report to the president. Under them are a series of vice presidents. At one site alone, we have ten vice presidents. Over me is the vice president of nursing. Under her are four directors. Under them are the nurse managers. Under the nurse managers are clinical nurse coordinators, and then staff nurses.

Can you imagine? You've got to go from the nurse to the nurse coordinator to the nurse manager to the director to the vice president of nursing to the COO to the CEO and then to the president. No wonder we are in hell. When you think about the information flow—they are always centralizing or decentral- izing—they don't know where they are, they don't know what they are doing or what anyone else does. It's amazing we can function at all.

When Maureen started at the hospital, in 1964, there was an ad- ministrator. There was also one person in finance, and there was a di- rector who reported to him. That changed as times got better and more money was produced:

As times got better, things got more complicated. We added a vice president for marketing, a vice president for finance, a vice president for services, a vice president for nursing, a vice president for purchasing, and a vice president for communications. We started adding so many vice presidents that it was hard to keep track. And under each vice president there was a departmental director.

I personally believe that incompetence starts at the vice presidential level. They are so tied into money that they do stupid things. Last year, all the vice presidents went to Vail, Colorado, to talk about cutting budgets. Their spouses accompanied them.

When they came back, their credibility took a hit. After all, how can you go to Vail and spend big dollars and then come back and recommend cutting an orderly?

Diving for Dollars

In 1993, Graef Crystal, an expert on executive compensation from the University of California at Berkeley, testified before a U.S. House of Representatives Subcommittee that the average pay for a chief executive in a healthcare-related company is $2.9 million—more than 85 times what a nurse makes. In addition, the CEO may receive stock options, cars, entertainment allowances, and other fringe benefits. Many of the women interviewed for this book stated that hospital directors, vice presidents, and CEOs get their share of perks, too. The perks, no doubt, offset the wear-and-tear of the job. The rationale given by many institutions is that individuals in highly visible jobs are more exposed to litigation and need something extra for the risks they take. That's a tough one to explain to women (and men) who daily risk infectious diseases, injuries on the job, and lawsuits. Everyone today is vulnerable to lawsuits. Many nurses are now taking courses on dealing with litigation—as a plaintiff, a defendant, and a witness. Where are their perks—the clothing allowances, cars, entertainment budgets, and bonuses?

There are too many inequities in the system. In the past, physicians have demanded expensive equipment for very select and rare procedures. Equipment can cost hundreds of thousands of dollars, even millions. In California, for example, several hospitals have hyperbaric decompression chambers; it is common for people to go skindiving in the Pacific. But having a decompression chamber in northern Montana doesn't make a lot of sense. Nevertheless, in their drive for power and their desire to keep up with the Joneses, some doctors pressure hospitals to carry financial burdens that make little sense, economically or otherwise.

Diane, an admissions coordinator, is glad to be out of nursing management. She believes that general nursing is pretty streamlined, but that there is fat in other departments:

> Nursing is pretty lean. I suspect it will be made leaner. In other departments, there are a lot of management people; there could be some streamlining done there. In nursing, we have always bit the bullet and found out later that other departments haven't reduced their personnel. Any type of reform is scary right now; my job could be affected. After all, if you don't have a lot of admissions, you don't need to have someone coordinate the process.

Accountability Makes the Difference

In the past few years, I have worked with hundreds of women's healthcare centers. I can count on the fingers of one hand the number that have implemented some method of measuring how their programs affect the women in their communities and what their participants contribute to hospital revenues.

Many of the women who are directors of women's centers, and whom I have had the pleasure of working with, are geniuses in their marketing strategies and programming. Some have taken over existing programs. Others have created programs and events from scratch. One visionary, from San Diego's Sharp Memorial Hospital, is Beverly Weurding. She presents an incredible array of functions for women of all ages in the San Diego area. Every year, she creates an all-day program that attracts over one thousand participants and is literally the talk of the town. At the end of each event, including the annual program, participants are surveyed about what, *exactly*, they want to see presented in the future. This feedback is critical and allows for fine-tuning. It's called *customer service*.

Some hospitals have empowered the directors of women's centers to join forces with other hospitals. In Kansas City, Jill Gerlach, with the Center for Women's Health at Shawnee Mission Medical Center, and Kristy Montgomery, with the Women's Resource Center at St. Luke's Hospital, have created their own separate programs that tie in with their respective hospitals' areas of expertise. Together, they have taken the next step: they have created an annual event by pooling their financial resources, staffs, and skills, and they have a great time doing it. As a dynamic duo, they are able to offer their communities innovative and timely topics.

These women and many like them have brought their vision and their touch to the workplace. They have made a significant difference to the women in their outreach areas. To continue offering their vision and their voices, they have developed methods of measuring their own effectiveness—and so must others. The majority of health-care decisions are made by women today, and women's health programs are viable businesses.

For women's centers and programs, one of the most critical tasks in changing times is to create measurement systems that will validate their position in hospitals. In other words, women's centers must view themselves as businesses, with standard profit-and-loss statements. It's the bottom line that counts.

Just Rewards

In locations that don't need decompression chambers, and where there are multiple types of visible inequities, it's easy to welcome change. Many women in nursing express heightened fear and stress in the workplace. Most of this stress seems to have resulted from physicians' fear of the coming changes in healthcare. Here is what Mary Ellen, a nurse manager, has to say:

> I don't know a nurse manager here who hasn't had a problem with
> a physician in the last couple of months. It seems that any little

thing will set them off. They complain about the most ridiculous things you can imagine.

Many of us believe that the physicians have been on the gravy train for a long time. In some places, they have actually bankrupted the system. We also believe that they are taking advantage of consumers. There is inequity in reimbursements, in terms of who works hard to provide care for patients.

I personally believe that it has been this self-centered approach in medicine that has literally corrupted our system. I feel it has to change, but I fear that it won't change in the right direction.

Mary Ellen believes that the physicians will be the last ones to suffer, because they still have power and prestige, and they control the purse-strings.

When it comes to who does the most work, some patients seem to agree with Mary Ellen, according to three studies. The studies show that when nurses are allowed to do their jobs properly, patients benefit. George Washington University did a study in 1986, showing that death rates in various intensive-care units were best predicted by just one factor: the level of nursing care. In 1990, a national study commissioned by Nurses of America, a consortium of nursing organizations, found that nurses far outshine other medical personnel in patients' minds: 77 percent of the respondents said that nurses played a constructive role in healthcare, compared with only 42 percent saying the same about doctors. And a study from Strong Memorial Hospital, in New York, showed that patients had a three times greater risk of dying or being readmitted into intensive care when doctors ignored nurses' suggestions.[1]

When it comes to the pursestrings, however, the women physicians did not agree with Mary Ellen. But why should they? Few of them are really in the powerful positions that their male colleagues have enjoyed for decades.

Margaret, a family-practice physician, feels that many doctors get a bad rap, and that many of them aren't in medicine for the money. Rather, they are there to help people:

> I hear lots of anger and depression, but I don't hear many ideas. Many of the doctors feel unappreciated. They feel like everyone is after them, that no one appreciates the work that is done. Despite what many say, most of us are not in medicine for the money.

Margaret believes that any type of change or reform in healthcare could be a disaster for doctors in general. She feels that doctors should not be construed as the culprits. There are others—namely, hospitals and attorneys.

Throughout the nineties, television, radio, and the print media have focused on reform in healthcare. Everyone knows that changes are coming, and the total impact will take years to evaluate. NBC's "Today" show did a segment on doctors' salaries, stating that the average was $190,000 a year. That generated a strong reaction from Margaret:

> That's just not true, at least not in my field. The show continued to say that doctors make too much money and ought to be regulated. My reaction to that is, when they regulate lawyers, they can regulate doctors.

Change, Change, Change

To survive and grow in a changing environment, whether professional or personal, takes a personal action plan. Change doesn't wait until you are ready to deal with it. It just happens, and quickly. The sooner you acknowledge it, the sooner you will be able to become an active participant in whatever the change is.

As change evolves, it's important to position yourself. Begin by making a commitment to continual improvement and to learning new things. Start a program that either enhances the current skills you have or expands them, and let them take you into another field.

There is no question that jobs are being eliminated as you read this. Windows close, but new doors open. Thousands and even millions of new products, jobs, and companies are created because of change. Inpatient care has shifted to outpatient care. In the past, insurance companies, the government, and even the medical community resisted home care (or at least paying for it), but that is changing, too.

Dramatic shifts in attitudes have emerged in the 1990s. New professions will open, expanding opportunities for nurses, technicians, doctors, and consultants serving this market. No longer will around-the-clock patient care be the norm; rather, patients and clients will need to hear all their instructions clearly in ten to twenty minutes. This means that greater communication skills are urgently needed by care providers. From that mere fact, gadgets and gimmicks will be produced and marketed to the home-care industry—items to trigger memory, facilitate care, and make life easier.

The evolving healthcare field must reinvent itself. It is and will continue to be one of the most important sectors of the economy. Embracing change enables you to take advantage of any opportunity that comes your way, so you won't be left behind.

Years ago, Helen Keller wrote,

> Security is mostly superstition. It does not exist in nature, nor do children of men (and women) as a whole, experience it. Avoiding danger is no safer in the long run than outright exposure. Life is either a daring adventure or nothing.

Change is inevitable. In order to exist and grow in today's world, you need to accept the fact that change surrounds you. If you will allow it, change will deliver phenomenal opportunities. The elimination of old habits and comfort zones will be celebrated. And that's exciting. Tomorrow truly will be another day.

16

Empowerment: The New Horizon

When women are empowered, they have the tools to give themselves permission to accomplish and succeed on their own. Empowering means enabling, authorizing, permitting, and giving power to—you give yourself the green light to pursue your personal vision.

Empowerment is not to be taken lightly. It's not a right, nor does it happen overnight. The women doctors who were interviewed for this book said that when they began to take steps that would empower their staff, everyone got along better.

When Joanie Jones first went to work in radiation oncology, she worked for Katherine Chapman, a woman physician who changed the way Joanie thought about work. Joanie said that Katherine was one of the first people she had ever come across who really believed in empowering women. She didn't spend a lot of time talking about it, but her actions spoke volumes:

> She would tell us about her education as a young woman training to be a doctor. At that time, in a class of one-hundred, ninety-nine would be men. She'd have no one to go have coffee with or have lunch with. She told us how the men would catch a cab and leave

her standing on the street. All the while this was being done to her, she would tell herself, "I will change this." And she did. She changed the work environment for us. Not only did she say, "I will help patients" but she said, "I will make sure you see that you can be more than you are."

When women move from sabotage to support, they move from helplessness to empowerment. With empowerment, you lead a significant and productive life, both personally and professionally. Empowerment is declaring, asserting and even demanding the right to be your true and authentic self. Within a group, empowerment requires a commitment from each member that enables all members to use collective strengths, abilities, and assets as resources. True empowerment will not exist unless there is an environment that allows and encourages the distribution of power. The development of your empowerment requires the roots of attention, belief, commitment, daring, and esteem.

When you pay *attention* to who you are, what you are, where you want to go, and what your options are for getting there, you are able to focus on your vision, your quest. Too often, a woman will spend time on activities that have nothing to do with what her vision is. This doesn't mean that you can't try new things or get involved in other ventures. It does mean that you say no to things and people who are draining, create negativity, and firehose your enthusiasm. When you pay attention, you support your decisions, your values, and your passions. Out of attention come growth and wisdom.

When you believe in yourself, you are able to hear that little voice—your conscience—that continually reaffirms and supports your authenticity, your mission, and your vision. It's easy to stand up and be counted, to speak up and speak out, when you have *belief* in yourself.

When you know who you are and believe in yourself, it's quite easy to stand up and say, "I am what I am, I believe in what I can do, and I have made a *commitment* to enabling myself, rather than waiting for permission from someone else." Your esteem for yourself is a critical ingredient in developing empowerment. The degree to which you value yourself, care about yourself, and regard yourself is directly related to your confidence. The greater it is, the more comfortable you are with yourself and others. With it, you will speak out and behave more assertively.

Women who have *daring* identify goals, create visions, and take risks, often huge ones. When you are daring, you allow yourself to experience the school of hard knocks, to make mistakes and fail. The woman who dares knows that when she hits a pothole, she will be able to climb out smarter and wiser—that she will grow with a changing workplace, not against it.

Actress Katharine Hepburn's mother gave her sound advice: "If you always do what interests you, then at least one person is pleased." Being empowered enables you to do what pleases you. As you earn your way toward empowerment, you become who you can be, honoring yourself and others.

One of the dark sides of the healthcare professions is that there are too many women who are deceitful, manipulative, conniving, and even vicious. Low self-esteem, inferiority, anxiety, doubt, fear, envy, and jealousy all play a critical part in the damage that women sometimes do to other women. Through empowerment, problems are identified and resolved. By committing yourself to solving them, you admit that they are there. You make a conscious effort to take responsibility for your own part in them, and you implement the changes necessary for eliminating them.

With empowerment, old taboos are revealed, discussed, and broken. Saying that women undermine other women has been taboo for too long. Your awareness, your commitment, and your courage to change old ways and behavior will bring a new day to working women. For an empowered woman, anything is possible.

Recommended Readings

Bright, D. *Criticism in Your Life.* New York: MasterMedia, 1988.

Buccholz, S. *Creating the High-Performance Team.* New York: Wiley, 1987.

Covey, S. *The Seven Habits of Highly Effective People.* New York: Simon & Schuster, 1989.

Deal, T. E., and Kennedy, A. A. *Corporate Cultures.* Reading, Mass.: Addison-Wesley, 1982.

Dowling, C. *Perfect Women.* New York: Summit Books, 1988.

Eichenbaum, L., and Orbach, S. *Between Women.* New York: Viking Penguin, 1988.

Forward, S. *Toxic Parents: Overcoming Their Hurtful Legacy and Reclaiming Your Life.* New York: Bantam Books, 1989.

French, M. *Beyond Power: On Women, Men, and Morals.* New York: Ballantine, 1985.

French, M. *The War Against Women.* New York: Summit Books, 1992.

Gray, J. *Men Are from Mars, Women Are from Venus.* New York: HarperCollins, 1982.

Handley, J., and Handley, R. *Why Women Worry.* Englewood Cliffs, N.J.: Prentice-Hall, 1990.

Harragan, B. L. *Games Mothers Never Taught You.* New York: Rawson Associates, 1977.

Helgesen, S. *The Female Advantage: Women's Ways of Leadership.* New York: Doubleday, 1990.

Hyatt, C. *Shifting Gears.* New York: Simon & Schuster, 1990.

Hyatt, C., and Gottlieb, L. *When Smart People Fail.* New York: Simon & Schuster, 1993.

Jackman, M. *Star Teams, Key Players.* New York: Holt, Rinehart & Winston, 1991.

Jeffers, S. *Feel the Fear and Do It Anyway.* New York: Random House, 1988.

Jeffries, E. N. *The Heart of Leadership.* Dubuque, Iowa: Kendall/Hunt, 1993.

Jongeward, D., and Scott, D. *Women as Winners.* Reading, Mass.: Addison-Wesley, 1983.

Kaminer, W. *I'm Dysfunctional, You're Dysfunctional.* Reading, Mass.: Addison-Wesley, 1992.

Kreigel, R. J. *If it ain't broke . . . BREAK IT!* New York: Warner Books, 1991.

Leonard, G. *Mastery.* New York: Dutton, 1991.

Lerner, H. G. *The Dance of Anger.* New York: HarperCollins, 1990.

Lerner, H. G. *The Dance of Deception.* New York: HarperCollins, 1993.

Loden, M. *Feminine Leadership, or How to Succeed in Business Without Being One of the Boys.* New York: Random House, 1985.

Madden, T. R. *Women Versus Women: The Uncivil Business War.* New York: AMACOM, 1987.

Marone, N. *Women and Risk: A Guide to Overcoming Learned Helplessness.* New York: St. Martin's Press, 1992.

Marshall, J. *Women Managers: Travelers in a Male World.* New York: Wiley, 1984.

McNally, M., and Schneider, P. *Hot Health Care Careers.* New York: MasterMedia, 1993.

Miller, J. B. *Toward a New Psychology of Women.* Boston: Beacon Press, 1976.

Moir, A., and Jessel, D. *Brain Sex: The Real Difference Between Men and Women.* New York: Lyle Stuart, 1991.

Morrison, A. M., White, R. P., and Velsorand, E. V. *Breaking the Glass Ceiling.* Reading, Mass.: Addison-Wesley, 1987.

Popcorn, F. *The Popcorn Report.* New York: Doubleday, 1992.

Rosener, J., and Loden, M. *Workforce America.* Homewood, Ill.: Dow Jones–Irwin, 1991.

Sanford, L. T., and Donovan, M. E. *Women and Self-Esteem.* New York: Viking Penguin, 1984.

Schaef, A. W. *Women's Reality.* Minneapolis: Winston Press, 1985.

Schapiro, N. *Negotiating for Your Life.* New York: Holt, Rinehart & Winston, 1993.

Schwartz, F. *Breaking with Tradition.* New York: Warner Books, 1992.

Scott, G. G. *Resolving Conflict.* Berkeley, Calif.: New Harbinger Publications, 1990.

Shames, K. H. *The Nightingale Conspiracy.* New York: Power Publications, 1993.

Shapiro, J. *Men: A Translation for Women.* New York: Viking Penguin, 1992.

Summers, C. *Caregiver, Caretaker.* Mt. Shasta, Calif.: Commune-a-Key Publishing, 1992.

Tavris, C. *The Mismeasure of Women.* New York: Simon & Schuster, 1992.

Teal, J., and Schneider, P. *Straight Talk on Women's Health.* New York: MasterMedia, 1993.

Walker, L. *The Battered Woman.* New York: HarperCollins, 1979.

Webb, S. L., *Shockwaves.* New York: MasterMedia, 1994.

Webb, S. L., *Step Forward: Sexual Harassment in the Workplace.* New York: Master Media, 1991.

Witken, G. *The Female Stress Syndrome.* Austin, Tex.: New Market Press, 1991.

Zeiger, C. A., and Allen, S. *Doing It All Isn't Everything.* Austin, Tex.: New Perspectives Press, 1992.

Notes

Chapter Two

1. K. Pennar and E. Mervosh, "Women at Work" (*Business Week*, Jan. 28, 1985), p. 80.

2. S. J. Diamond, "Women on the Job: Surge Widely Felt" (*Los Angeles Times*, Sept. 9, 1984), p. 80.

3. M. D. Naylor and M. B. Sherman, "Nurses for the Future. Wanted: The Best and the Brightest" (*American Journal of Nursing, 87, 12*), pp. 1601–1605.

4. L. Gasparis Vonfrolio and J. Swirsky, *Nurse Abuse: Impact and Resolution* (New York: Power Publications, 1993).

5. Gasparis Vonfrolio and Swirksy, *Nurse Abuse.*

6. Diamond, "Women on the Job."

7. H. Rogan, "Women Executives Feel That Men Both Aid and Hinder Their Careers" (*Wall Street Journal*, Oct. 29, 1984), p. 31.

8. P. Krueger, "What Women Think of Women Bosses" (*Working Woman*, June 1993), pp. 40–41.

9. P. Berger, "Battered Pillars of the American System" (*Fortune*, Apr. 1975), pp. 133–150.

10. T. J. Hayes, "Ethics in Business: Problem Identification and Potential Solutions" (*Hospital Material Management Quarterly*, May 1983), pp. 37–38.

11. D. F. Linowes, "International Business and Morality" (address delivered to the Center for International Education, Urbana–Champaign, Ill., March 25, 1977).

12. R. M. Kanter, *Men and Women of the Corporation* (New York: Basic Books, 1977), pp. 77, 82, 134.

13. Kanter, *Men and Women of the Corporation.*
14. Kanter, *Men and Women of the Corporation,* p. 151.
15. Kanter, *Men and Women of the Corporation,* p. 158.
16. Kreuger, "What Women Think of Women Bosses."
17. Kreuger, "What Women Think of Women Bosses," pp. 40–43.
18. Kreuger, "What Women Think of Women Bosses," pp. 40–43.
19. J. Briles, *Woman to Woman: From Sabotage to Support* (Far Hills, N.J.: Horizon Press), pp. 32–36.
20. Briles, *Woman to Woman.*
21. C. Gilligan, *In a Different Voice* (Cambridge, Mass.: Harvard University Press, 1982), p. 10.
22. Briles, *Woman to Woman,* pp. 37–38.
23. J. Trotesky, "Must Women Executives Be Such Barracudas?" (*Wall Street Journal,* Nov. 9, 1981), p. 24.
24. G. W. Bowman, N. B. Worthy, and S. A. Greyser, "Are Women Executives People?" (*Harvard Business Review,* July–August 1965), pp. 95–101.
25. C. A. Beauvais, "The Family and the Work Group: Dilemmas for Women in Authority" (*Dissertation Abstracts International,* 1977, *37*), p. 3595-B.
26. A. Hochschild, *Second Shift* (New York: Viking, 1989).
27. H. Rogan, "Executive Women Find It Difficult to Balance Demands on the Job, Home" (*Wall Street Journal,* Oct. 30, 1984), p. 33.
28. J. Briles, *The Confidence Factor* (New York: MasterMedia, 1990).
29. "Living in a Man's World . . . and Not Turning into a Man" (*Vogue,* Aug. 1993), p. 301.
30. M. Bayes and P. Newton, "Women in Authority: A Sociophysiological Analysis" (*Journal of Applied Behavioral Science,* 1978, *14*), p. 9.
31. Bayes and Newton, "Women in Authority," p. 14.
32. Bayes and Newton, "Women in Authority," p. 17.
33. Bayes and Newton, "Women in Authority," pp. 18–20.
34. C. D. Sutton and K. K. Moore, "Executive Women—Twenty Years Later" (*Harvard Business Review,* Sept.–Oct. 1985), p. 2.

Chapter Six

1. V. M. Farley, "How to Get What We Deserve" (*Revolution: The Journal of Nurse Empowerment,* Spring 1992), p. 25.
2. Letter to the editor (*Revolution: The Journal of Nurse Empowerment,* Spring 1992), p. 9.

3. B. Buresh, "Media Watch" (*Revolution: The Journal of Nurse Empowerment*, Spring 1992), p. 14.

4. Buresh, "Media Watch."

5. Buresh, "Media Watch."

Chapter Ten

1. M. Jackman, *Star Teams, Key Players* (Troy, Mo.: Holt, Rinehart & Winston, 1991), p. 5.

2. Jackman, *Star Teams, Key Players*, p. 6.

Chapter Thirteen

1. S. L. Webb, *Step Forward: Sexual Harassment in the Workplace* (New York: MasterMedia, 1991), pp. 25–29.

2. Webb, *Step Forward*, pp. 25–29.

3. D. Q. Haney, "Interns Cite Sexual Harassment" (*Denver Post*, Feb. 4, 1993).

4. Webb, *Step Forward*, pp. 94–101.

Chapter Fourteen

1. P. Kreuger, "What Women Think of Women Bosses" (*Working Woman*, June 1993), p. 41.

2. J. W. Driscoll, *Mentoring in Nursing* (Philadelphia: Wyeth-Ayerst Laboratories, 1993). For information on obtaining this video, write to the company at P.O. Box 8299, Philadelphia, PA 19101, or call (215) 971-5872. Another useful resource on mentoring is *The Pocket Mentor*, published by the Association of Women Surgeons. To purchase a copy ($15), write to the association at 414 Plaza Drive, Suite 209, Westmont, IL 60559, or call (708) 655-0392.

Chapter Fifteen

1. "Bouquets" (*Boston Globe*, April 2, 1992).

The Author

JUDITH BRILES is the founder of The Briles Group, Inc., and the author of ten other books, including: *Woman to Woman; The Confidence Factor; The Workplace; When God Says NO; Financial Savvy for Women;* and *The Dollars and Sense of Divorce.* She earned her M.B.A. degree from Pepperdine University (1980) and her Ph.D. degree in business administration from Nova University (1990). Her clients include hospitals, medical centers, and healthcare professional associations in the United States and Canada. She is a past director of the National Speakers' Association and the Colorado Women's Leadership Coalition. She also serves on the advisory boards of the Miss America Pageant, *Colorado Women News,* and the Colorado League of Nursing. She is the first honorary member of the Association of Women Surgeons.

For information on Judith Briles's speeches, workshops, cruises designed for healthcare professionals, and her newsletter, *The Woman's Voice,* please contact her at:

The Briles Group, Inc.
P.O. Box 22021
Denver, CO 80222
(303) 745-4590 or (303) 745-4595 FAX

Index

REVOLUTION—The Journal of Nurse Empowerment, 103
Ruane, B., 139
Rules. *See* Unwritten rules

S

Sabotage: actions of, 57–58; costs of, 10–13; by co-workers, 81–109; denial of, 26–27; and friendships, 19–21; and gender, 9–10, 14–16, 17–19; incidence of, 21–22; by mentor, 229; and motivation for work, 13–14; quiz on, 49–56; reasons for, of women by women, 24–26; respondents to survey on, 4–6; and support, 16–17; survey findings on, 6–9; by unwritten rules, 164–170; in workplace, 58–79
Saboteurs: survey findings on, 14; on teams, 185–187
Salary: confrontation over, 147–148; of doctors, 240; of healthcare executives, 236; men's versus women's, 27; and self-esteem, 46–47; of women in healthcare, 24
Schroeder, P., 132
Scott, G. G., 118
Secretaries: power identification by, 36; women as, 29
Self-esteem, and salary, 46–47
Sexual harassment: blaming victim in, 218; combatting, 212; dealing with complaints of, 219; description of, 208–210; harassers in, 216, 218–219; in medicine, 211–212, 214; physician's speaking up about, 131–133; tips for employees on, 220–223; tips for supervisors on, 223–224; types of, 210–211; victims in, 214–215; victim trap in, 217–218; by women, 212–214

Shared governance, 104
Speaking up, 129–130; case studies of, 130–138; to media, 130–131, 138–139; on teams, 179–180
Stereotypes: holding women back, 25–26; and work by women, 31–32
Substance abuse, speaking up about, 134–135
Supervisors. *See* Managers
Survey of 1987, 3–4, 6, 7–8, 9, 11, 14, 15, 21–22
Survey of 1993: on costs of sabotage, 10–13; on differences in women and men, 9–10; findings from, 6–9; on friendships, 19–21; on gender, 15–16, 17–19; on motivation for work, 13–14; respondents to, 4–6; on saboteurs, 14; on support, 16–17; on unethical behavior, 21–22
Sutton, C. D., 48–49

T

Team player, 171–172
Teams, 171–173; case histories of women on, 174–184; development phases of, 173–174; handling annoyances and attitudes on, 184–185; identifying saboteurs on, 185–187; unwritten rules about, 158–159
Television. *See* Media
Thatcher, M., 118
Tiwanak, G., 106
Trotesky, J., 43
Trust, broken, 92–95

U

Unethical behavior, 4. *See also* Sabotage
Unwritten rules, 154–155; breaking, 164–170; circulating, 170; identifying, 162–164; sample, 156–162